Contents

IEA Health and Welfare Unit

Health Unit Paper No. 8

MEDICAL CARE: IS IT A CONSUMER GOOD?

Medical Care: Is It A Consumer Good?

**Brendan Devlin, Michael Freeman, Iain Hanham,
James Le Fanu, Robert Lefever, Brian Mantell**

London
The IEA Health and Welfare Unit
1990

First published in March 1990
by
The IEA Health and Welfare Unit
2 Lord North St
London SW1P 3LB

© The IEA Health and Welfare Unit 1990

ISBN 0-255 36258-7

Typeset by the IEA Health and Welfare Unit
Printed in Great Britain by
Goron Pro-Print Co. Ltd
Churchill Industrial Estate, Lancing, West Sussex

Foreword

Is medical care different from other consumer goods? How much medical care is pure science, and how much more like an art? How much room is there for reasonable differences of view about methods of treatment and whether or not to treat at all? And how much room is there for consumer choice based on informed consent?

During the last couple of years there has been an intense debate about the future of the NHS and in particular about the extent to which there should be greater competition. The dispute between 'command' and 'market' approaches to the NHS rests primarily on assumptions about the nature of medical decision making. Supporters of the traditional NHS incline to the view that medical treatment is in the nature of a necessity or need, whereas advocates of market competition believe that medical treatment is more akin to a consumer good.

The view that medical care is a need leads to the conclusion that health care should be an absolute priority in the allocation of government funds. Consequently the assumption that underlies much medical debate is that everything that medically can be done should be done and money should be no object. Two assumptions lie behind this attitude. The first is that health care is like emergency care — at least urgent and possibly a matter of life and death. People have in mind accidents and severe or sudden illness. The second assumption is that medicine is primarily scientific.

There are counter views to both assumptions. Although much public debate proceeds as if health care was like emergency care, the reality is that the NHS provides a diverse range of services many of which are not urgent. And in practice, despite their rhetoric, governments of all parties have recognised that the NHS provides many services which are not absolute priorities. They may be desirable but not necessarily more desirable than the many other good things which governments are expected to finance from taxes. Most people regard their own health in much the same way. They see good health as desirable but not an absolute priority, as smoking, eating and drinking behaviour testifies.

The popular belief that medicine is a largely scientific endeavour is no less resilient, but most doctors would acknowledge that medicine is as much an art as a science. A good deal of medical intervention is based on trial-and-error rather than on strict scientific evaluation and many would argue that this is inevitably so.

Yet, these realities have not fully permeated day to day debate about the future of the NHS. We have, therefore, invited four distinguished NHS consultants and two GPs to reflect on the character of medical practice by drawing primarily on examples from their own experience. They each offer new insights into the dilemmas, uncertainties and complexities of medical practice.

Health care is not unitary. It embraces a diverse range of personal services, about which there is much room for personal preference. This has two main implications. First, contrary to the claims of some health economists, professional expertise is not so impregnable that consumer sovereignty is an impossibility. There is an important role for informed consumer choice.

Second, because health care is partly a matter of personal preference, the government has no way of determining the correct or optimal amount to spend on the NHS. It also means that if the government continues to try to finance health care from taxation it will discover that there is no sum of money it can spend which will satisfy public expectations without also creating a fiscal crisis. Without awareness of prices and the alternatives that must be foregone in order to consume desirable but non-essential medical services, public expectations will always outpace any government's ability to raise taxes to meet medical demand.

Finally, may I thank the authors for participating in this project. Their essays are admirably frank about the difficult choices and the imponderables faced by doctors. We have come a long way from the days of medical mystique. None of the authors necessarily shares the conclusions I have drawn and some are strongly committed to the NHS. It is, therefore, very much to their credit that they have put the professional duty to educate and inform above short-run partisan loyalties. It also goes without saying that no one else connected with the IEA necessarily shares the views expressed in this paper but it is published as a timely and informative contribution to public debate about the future of health care in Britain.

David G. Green

Part 1

Reflections from Provincial Surgical Practice 1989

H. Brendan Devlin

The Author

Brendan Devlin is a member of the Council of the Royal College of Surgeons of England, a Lecturer in Clinical Surgery at the University of Newcastle upon Tyne and a Consultant Surgeon at North Tees General Hospital, Stockton-on-Tees. He is the Secretary of the National Confidential Enquiry into Perioperative Deaths and the author or co-author of numerous books and scientific articles on surgery and allied topics.

1

Reflections from
Provincial Surgical Practice 1989

'Consumerism', 'market forces', 'quality assurance' and 'competition' are new threatening words ill understood by most British doctors. Although these concepts are relevant to daily living for the man in the street, many of my medical colleagues do not perceive their relevance to medical practice. Since 1948, the corporate National Health Service has allowed British medicine to become progressively more remote from the everyday commercial and social life of the United Kingdom. Periodically problems within the NHS have brought doctors into political controversy, usually over funding issues, and campaigns generated by doctors have changed everyday life; helmets for motorcyclists and seat belts are good examples.

However, despite these forays into wider public life, medicine has remained a self contained profession managed by ancient and respectable institutions. There is no flow of new personnel into medicine throughout a working life; once in medicine people do not readily abandon it as a career and there is no inflow of new recruits from among the mature workforce who have other industrial experience. The majority of our recruits come from a very similar background, most are direct from secondary school, all are required to present with 'science' A levels: school chemistry, school physics and school biology are the last non-vocational inputs these young people are subjected to. Then there is the hermetically closed medical school education which occupies five years grappling with a curriculum overloaded with the rote learning of the facts of every specialism in medicine. There is now so much medicine for the medical student to learn that we can hardly find space to squeeze in the behavioural sciences, economics and political awareness that all other university students acquire by leisure time osmosis on their multidisciplinary campuses. Medicine, like medieval monasticism, has become a state apart from national life.

Consumerism

'Consumerism' is a recent word in English. It connotes choice for the provider to market a particular product and choice for the consumer to purchase it. The word 'consumerism' causes antibodies in many consultant colleagues who do not perceive medicine as a commodity to be sold off the shelf like tins of beans.

Applied to contemporary medicine 'consumerism' has conflicting meanings. From the funder's perspective, how far is the medical market driven by consumer demand and how far is it driven by clinical/pathological factors beyond the consumer's control? Is medicine subject to the day-to-day discipline of the market place?

From the patient's (consumer's) perspective the issue is choice, choice of family practitioner, of consultant, of hospital, of admission date, etc. Thus there is choice of which supermarket to go to and when to visit the store, but the choice exercised within the store is not applicable to medicine. The choice available in the supermarket does not operate, patients do not choose between a heart transplant and a knee replacement as they choose between smoked salmon or kippers in the store. None the less there is some consumer choice, one patient will choose to have her varicose veins treated surgically, another will not.

We need to understand the extent of this customer choice if we are to redefine the UK system into a consumerist paradise either with or without independently funded elements. Within the UK the vast majority of hospital in-patients and those in nursing homes and other residential units are the elderly and the psychologically ill. Choice and consumerism do not figure on their sad agenda. Within the acute sector, patients in beds in all the medical specialties — general medicine, cardiology, neurology, nephrology, gastroenterology, etc. — are always those with acute illness requiring urgent investigation or management. Looking at our own microsystem in Stockton-on-Tees, 95 per cent of all medical specialty admissions are emergencies taken in urgently with life or limb threatening conditions. Within the surgical disciplines 50 per cent overall are emergency admissions (Table 1). In surgical disciplines the range is from 45 per cent emergencies in general surgery to 60 per cent emergencies in orthopaedics. Many of the non-emergency admissions in surgical disciplines are also patients with life-threatening diseases, cancer and vascular disease being the big problems in general surgery. Of the 5,077 general surgical admissions to our service in 1989 only 478 (9 per cent) were patients having elective surgery for non-life threatening diseases. With these figures it is easy to understand how provincial consultants are sceptical of the supermarket concept of health care.

Outside London and the bigger conurbations there is usually only one supplier of specialist medical services in each town - — the local district general hospital — hence patients cannot exercise much choice. Even were choice available to travel to the next town or elsewhere for treatment, a voucher system for instance, those requiring treatment most frequently are the elderly and the less well to do in society, not population groups with great consumerist muscle.

Table 1
Admissions to North Tees General Hospital Over the Year Ending 31 March 1989

	Available Beds	Admissions		Day Cases		Total	% Non Elective
		Elective	Non-elective	Elective	Non-elective		
Mental Illness	115	-	656	-	-	656	100
Elderly Care	176	-	1867	-	1	1868	100
General Medicine	115	-	4487	-	1085	5572	100
General Surgery*	91	1816	2697	1297	167	5977	45
Trauma & Orthopaedics	66	557	1233	338	82	2210	40
Paediatrics	32	-	1429	-	32	1461	100
Gynaecology	31	1568	1327	90	122	3107	47
Other Specialties	142	232	5012	77	204	5525	94
TOTALS	**768**	**4173**	**18708**	**1802**	**1693**	**26376**	**77**

*NOTE: Including urology; only 9% were patients having elective surgery for non-life threatening conditions.

Market Forces

It is often opined that long waiting lists and excessive waiting times for clinics are characteristics of the centrally managed bureaucratic NHS and that the adoption of a market orientation would alleviate this.

Waiting lists for surgery are a problem. Why they exist in some districts and not in others is a baffling social phenomenon. Firstly, it is not true to say they don't exist in more market-orientated health care systems; anyone who has worked as a junior doctor resident in the USA will recount the end-stage patients admitted to American university hospitals, patients who avoided consulting a doctor when their condition was reversible and curable because they could not afford the cost. So there is a hidden waiting list problem in the USA and we do not want the social and personal consequences of that system imported into Britain.

Part of the waiting list problem is the success of modern medicine accentuated in the UK by the system of financing the NHS. Again, in our microsystem in Stockton-on-Tees over the 19 years since I became a consultant, the output from the Department of General Surgery has increased from 3,301 patients treated in 1969 to 5,977 patients treated in 1988, an increase of over 80 per cent (Table 2). Because of the curious method of funding the district hospital this increased productivity is not reflected by any additional revenue; in fact, although we were doing better the district was effectively worse off! So cost restraint has stopped us doing more!

Table 2
General Surgery Admissions
to North Tees General Hospital 1969-1988

	Admissions
1969	3,301
1974	3,498
1979	5,407
1984	5,855
1988	5,977

But waiting lists are a problem and a problem we should endeavour to solve. Waiting lists exist in general surgery, trauma and orthopaedic surgery, ENT surgery, gynaecology and ophthalmology (Table 3). The diagnosis categories of these patients are listed in Figure 1. Reviewing these diagnoses there is no doubt that cataract removal is a very worthwhile procedure giving instant sight back to elderly people. Hip replacement is worthwhile to increase the mobility of many elderly people with arthritis. Haemorrhoidectomy is an operation of doubtful value in many cases; the same goes for tonsils and adenoids and some varicose vein operations. Hernias are life-threatening if they obstruct and strangulate, particularly in the very young and the very old. The criteria for inclusion on a waiting list and the criteria for surgery need refining and making more explicit.

Table 3

Patients on Waiting Lists at 31 March 1987

	Number
General surgery	141,918
Traumatic & orthopaedic surgery	137,807
Ear, nose & throat surgery	104,535
Gynaecology	90,587
Ophthalmology	57,868

Figure 1

Diagnosis Categories of Patients on Waiting Lists at 31 March 1987

Cataract

Hip Replacements

Haemorrhoids

Inguinal Hernias

Tonsils & Adenoids

Varicose Veins

Clearly the waiting lists are a problem and some action is necessary on this front. As an immediate response the menu of what is offered on the NHS could be reviewed and any treatments not contributing to the health of the population removed. Rather like restricting prescribing to the generic drugs shown to have clinical value, surgical operations without defined clinical indications and benefits could be taken off the list, but this would not significantly alter the overall picture.

Another strategy is to offer incentives to surgeons to tackle waiting lists. There could be merit in this application of market forces; equally without adequate regulation it could distort the 'market' and prevent patients with more serious ailments achieving the priority they need.

A market strategy, direct from success in industry and the USA, is to encourage innovation. Day hospitals and hernia centres are highly successful American initiatives which the NHS has failed to develop. Funding has always been the problem to date. If funding just travelled with the patient there would be no problem. Simply paying those hospitals who do the work for what they do would work wonders. If our budget in Stockton-on-Tees had increased by the 80 per cent our productivity did from 1970 to 1988 'market forces' would have me as its apostle!

Quality Assurance

Both my profession and the public have come to believe that our interventions are inevitably beneficial and that the outcomes of our activities are guaranteed. This concept is encouraged by lawyers who seem able to sustain the argument that if intervention does not give a 100 per cent good outcome someone, usually the doctor, is at fault. This paradigm of acute medicine or surgery does not withstand the scrutiny that modern information technology and mathematical logic permits. The read-out of an encounter with a surgeon for an acute illness, say appendicitis, conventionally states medical history plus physical examination plus laboratory tests enable an accurate diagnosis: an operation should follow: the outcome is beyond question and excellent: some two weeks later the patient will be fit and well.

However, when each stage of this process is subjected to critical evaluation, flaws are discovered. Doctors only elicit 60 per cent of the correct history, doctors can overlook and misinterpret physical signs, and the clinical diagnosis of appendicitis is incorrect in about 50 per cent of cases when made by junior surgeons. Some 30-40 per cent of appendices removed in the United Kingdom do not show any evidence of acute appendicitis.[1] When we go on to review the resources used to treat appendicitis we uncover even greater variations in medical practice: for example the duration of stay in hospital for an appendix operation varies from 2 to 12 days and post-operative complications are recorded in up to 15 per cent of patients in some series.[2]

Variation in Outcome

Clinical medicine is a very uncertain science. Over the last 15 years or so the scrutiny of medical practice using today's computers has thrown up many discrepancies which have given us a jolt; a study in the 1970s showed that failure rates of intestinal joints (anastomoses) which were made when surgeons connected large bowel (colon) together after removing cancers varied from 3 to 30 per cent. The failure rate varied depending on which surgeon did the operation.[3] These 'operator dependent variables' could have significant bad results for all concerned. For the patient a leaking anastomosis would be followed by sepsis, abscesses and even death; for

---

[1] Hoffman, J., Rasmussen O., 'Aids in the Diagnosis of Acute Appendicitis', *British Journal of Surgery*, 1989, 76: 774-9.

[2] Morgan, M., Paul, E., Devlin, H.B., 'Length of Stay for Common Surgical Procedures: Variations among Districts'. *British Journal of Surgery*, 1987, 74: 884-9.

[3] Fielding, L.P., *et al.* 'Anastomotic Integrity after Operations for Large Bowel Cancer: A Multicentre Study', *British Medical Journal*, 1980, 281: 411-14.

the NHS a leaking anastomosis means a longer stay in hospital, the costs of antibiotics and re-operation in some cases.

There is no purpose in constructing a litany of this literature on the variability of medical practice here, but it is helpful to us to realise that more skilled and senior clinicians perform better than junior doctors and that there is a close relationship between the outcomes of surgery and the volume of operating for that condition performed by the surgeon. Put concisely, the specialist regularly doing the operation gets very much better results than the occasional operator.

Another factor related to outcome is the hospital, particularly its size and the organisation of the services within it. For example, it has been demonstrated that the outcome after prostatectomy, another very common surgical operation, is better if the operating surgeon is a skilled urologist who does many of the operations (the volume/outcome factor we have already mentioned) and if the patients undergoing the operation are grouped in a specialised (urology) ward within the hospital.[1]

From these rather dry observations on clinical practice we can, perhaps, draw some inferences for public and economic policy.

There is great merit in providing surgical services in special units so that the surgeons have an adequate workload to develop their skills. Furthermore, the outcomes of surgery are improved if the patients are concentrated in wards and units where nursing and other skills can be enhanced by constant practice and education. The case for further regionalising surgical services is powerful.[2] The parallel from industry cannot be overlooked; a well managed factory is more competitive

---

[1] Wennberg, J.E., et al., 'Use of Claims Data to Evaluate Health Care Outcomes: Mortality and Re-operation following Prostatectomy'. JAMA, 1987, 257: 933-6.

[2] Hannan, E.L., et al,. 'Investigation of the Relationship between Volume and Mortality for Surgical Procedures Performed in New York State Hospitals', JAMA, 1989, 262: 503-10.

than a cottage industry. With good quality control on the conveyer belt the customer is happier, too.

Quality control in medical and surgical practice by clinical audit, reviewing clinical activity and relaying the results of this review and recommendations arising therefrom to clinicians, has had an impact on practice and should have a great and more sustained impact in the future.

Until recently, large-scale review of clinical practice was not possible. Until user-friendly computing came along medical audit was a task undertaken only by enthusiasts with punch cards or ledgers. The innate conservatism of doctors also turned them off audit. However the climate of opinion is changing and *The Report of a Confidential Enquiry into Perioperative Deaths*, demonstrated that a fair appraisal of clinical activity could be carried out on a large scale by the profession.[1] It showed that this could be done without putting too great a burden on the individual, and that the results could be appraised by the profession and recommendations brought forward without damaging individual patients or doctors. Medical audit is here to stay. The problems are to improve its effectiveness and most importantly to define the objectives of medicine so that they can be measured mathematically.[2]

Competition

Competition is undoubtedly a regulator in commerce where alternative sources of supply can spring up but in medicine there is only one profession that can supply the service. Making doctors compete with each other is spurious competition if there is no adequate public regulation of the market. The scope for insider dealing to subvert competition within the medical profession is enormous. The in-built conservatism

[1] Buck, N., Devlin, H.B., Lunn, J.N., *The Report of a Confidential Enquiry into Perioperative Deaths*, London: The Nuffield Provincial Hospitals Trust/King's Fund, 1987.

[2] Devlin, H.B., 'Professional Audit, Quality Control and Keeping up to Date', *Bailliere's Clinical Anaesthesiology* 1988, 2: 299-324.

of the profession, plus its resources committed to its panoply of fissiparous corporate power, provide an in-built support for the status quo and are the most powerful anti-competition lobby within the UK today. There is a need for a wholesale rethink of the institutions of medicine, for a strong regulatory body with powerful non-medical input. The restructuring of medicine should be a higher priority than tinkering with the organisation of the NHS and all the political hazards that task includes, political hazards that are all too likely to be translated into votes. Reform of the institutions of medicine is unlikely to generate vast voter opposition and could unbungle the system without abandoning the concept of a National Health Service.

The Need for Facts

If British medicine is to respond to quality initiatives and subject itself to the priorities of market forces, information will be needed. Few people realise the inadequacy of the current NHS information system. Great studies have been made in recent years in improving the financial management information systems, but clinical information available on a global scale is still scarce and inexact. *The Report of a Confidential Enquiry into Perioperative Deaths*[1] demonstrated the failings of the information base the NHS was working on. It was difficult to establish how many doctors or consultants were employed, how many patients were treated and even how many deaths had occurred! For meaningful clinical audit to take place a massive investment in information technology will be needed. Even if the cash is available for this investment in hardware, we are still light years away from developing the software to undertake meaningful comparisons and costings between different clinical policies. We urgently need to make progress in this field. Writing and researching definitions of

---

[1] *Op. cit.*

clinical status, making values for clinical indicators of the medical process and developing outcome measures of medical intervention are skilled tasks that will consume much medical manpower, but they are tasks we must undertake urgently if our health care is to be improved and made more relevant.[1] Developing clinical information is a fascinating task. The application of computer logic to day-to-day clinical management, audit of outcome and patient satisfaction indices is an exciting prospect for medicine. If we could get the technology right and accessible in every clinical situation we could offer a brighter prospect for doctors and vastly improved care to patients. Computerised medicine should advance efficiency and effectiveness and equity of health care in the UK.

The Clinicians

My earlier disparaging comparisons between medicine as a cottage industry and managed medicine producing a consumer-desirable output should prompt reflection on the structure of hospital medical practice. The extant situation — consultant at the top and all consultants equal to each other, and then a hierarchy of aspirants from senior registrars, registrars, senior house officers to lowly house officers — should be reconsidered. This new thinking could start at either end of the pyramid. Why do consultants usually remain in one place once they are appointed? Are all consultants of equal value? If they are, why are some more prominent than others? Why do some contribute more than others? Why do some get merit and distinction awards when others don't? Are all senior registrars being constantly supervised and trained? Do we need all the punishing years of 'training' for our junior doctors in the UK before we allow them independent clinical practice? Other competitor nations don't have this dragged-out training career. Do we need all these junior doctors doing these horrendous

---

[1] Shaw, C.D., 'Clinical Outcome Indicators', *Health Trends*, 1989, 21: 37-9.

hours of duty? Some systems have far fewer resident doctor populations than we do. Could some simple, regular, routine tasks be turned into written orders and undertaken by non-medical personnel? Is working in shifts possible? These questions must be faced.

Nowadays patients are in hospital for a much shorter time than they were when many of the current consultants were in training. The patients are generally older and iller today. There are more possible interventions. It is no use my saying 'When I was a houseman...' because there were no intravenous antibiotics to give, no life support systems to manage, no transplants then! Medicine has changed and the structure of medicine needs to change, too.

Specialty Teams

Surely consultants should be grouped together as specialty teams for evaluation of their clinical outcomes and as cost centres for financial management? Then they could co-operate with each other and use consistent and congruent clinical policies; ones that could be written so that some routines could be downloaded to non-medical personnel. Work shifts so that there was always a consultant readily available?

The juniors must surely be admitted to the 20th century and allowed shorter hours, more realistic work patterns and perhaps taught rather than learning by osmosis. Junior doctors in the NHS suffer perhaps the worst working conditions in the EEC — house officers working 90-100 hours per week are not unusual. The consultants cannot agree among themselves how to share their work or adapt modern concepts of personnel management and skill to contemporary clinical practice so it is not surprising that consultants cling to the concept of 'their' registrar and 'their' houseman. Consultants are so badly organised coping with their patients 24 hours a day, doing emergency calls, etc., that the juniors are often left unsupervised. Consultants working in teams could share all this work. The idea of consultant teams or divisions brings us to leadership and incentives, both unspeakable in the present collectivist NHS.

Clinical Directors

Could there be clinical directors recruited by advertisement and competition from the consultant body? The clinical director would set and co-ordinate policy, establish quality review and be allowed to reward staff for what they do. Directors would have to be remunerated accordingly. If you chose preferment and proved yourself as a consultant you could apply for a clinical directorate elsewhere; this would allow consultants to move as their skills and capabilities changed. I stress the importance of clinical directors being appointed from 'elsewhere', as the 'buggins' turn' method of finding committee chairmen is the most fossilising factor in many British hospitals.

There is unmistakable evidence from studies in the USA, Canada and continental Europe that clinical activity and patient outcomes are related to consultant/senior clinician involvement in the hospital administration. In Britain since 1948 we have had 'administration' which has always seen itself, and been seen by clinicians, as separate from the medical and nursing activity. This separation reached its zenith in the era of consensus management from 1974 to 1982. General management has improved the situation but we still suffer from this dichotomy of purpose, so clinically led management is certainly the optimum we should strive to achieve.[1]

Regulation and the Institutions of Medicine

As medicine has pursued its own destiny, since 1948 cocooned from political and economic realities by the NHS, it has not significantly modernised its own institutions. Like the medieval monasteries abolished for economic reasons in 1536 the great

---

[1] Shortell, S.M., Logerfo, J.P., 'Hospital Medical Staff Organisation and the Quality of Care', *Medical Care*, 1981, 19: 1041-55.

medical institutions have 'reformed' themselves and begotten daughter houses, but they are reluctant to rethink their roles. Since the coming of the NHS the number of medical royal colleges has expanded and continues to increase faster and faster. Cynics believe that in perhaps five years time the sole function of the Privy Council will be providing Royal Charters to even more exotic subspecialism colleges of my profession! Each of these new colleges replicates its predecessors and provides yet another non-political site for the royals to visit with propriety.

Yet I'm at a loss to decide what this vital professional proliferation of separateness has achieved for the health of citizens in the UK.

The grand oversight of all the Brownian activity of medicine is vested in the General Medical Council, a body steeped in its late Victorian and Edwardian success but dominated from within medicine's own ranks. Self-regulation may be the hall-mark of a profession but surely this self-regulation should be in the public interest? How can you know the public interest if the public is excluded from the decision and policy-making process?

In a system when you have an almost monopoly funder of health care, the state through the NHS, and a monopoly supplier, the medical profession, there would seem to be a very cogent argument for a strong regulator in the public interest. The debate over British Telecom and water privatisation has a special relevance for medicine.

Sadly, to date no government has seemed anxious to address this medical corporatism. Governments recognise and benefit from the confusion and isolationism of organised medicine but they seem reluctant to promote, or indeed investigate, the internal state of medicine. A simple holding operation by the Privy Council to prevent the spawning of more medical institutions would be a start and a reluctance to sanction further medical charities might bring a cold wind of economic reality to blow away some cobwebs and cause a re-think.

If the medical profession is to retain its privileges it must be able to monitor and discipline doctors, retrain them if necessary and guarantee their competence if public confidence is to be retained. To respond to the challenges of the new technology and quality standards, the role of the Royal Colleges and the General Medical Council must be refined, consolidated and strengthened. This is as important as restructuring the management arrangements for our work. Currently any doctor on the British register can undertake any clinical activity: we have no universally applied criteria of specialisation and a confusing system of postgraduate medical education.[1] We need an examination/accreditation system that allows us to publish for the consumers a list of specialists in appropriate disciplines, identifying 'a surgeon' is not enough because medicine is too specialised today. We need a continuous monitoring process to ensure that specialists keep up to date and we need adequate quality control of practice. The consumer or patient needs to know this is effective. I regard these functions as very much within the province of the Medical Royal Colleges but they must be given a new legislative framework to be effective.

The introduction of an indicative medical register specifying who could practise unsupervised in each medical specialism would also allow us to review the content of the core medical undergraduate curriculum. No longer would the newly qualified doctor need to know a smattering of everything, or be allowed to practise every specialty unsupervised. Instead, the medical undergraduate curriculum could be shortened and thinned out, again allowing medical students to be educated. And, who knows? Encourage more mature persons to take up medicine as part of a career change. If we could reform the institutions of medicine and disentangle medical education the scope for reform is infinite.

---

[1] Dowie, R., *Postgraduate Medical Education and Training in the United Kingdom*, London: King's Fund, 1987.

If you are naive enough to see the institutions of medicine as medieval you will immediately recognise our work practices as serfdom securely based in *olde* English cottage industry cost centres clustered around the manor of this landscape, the local district general hospital. Unfortunately the landscape outside has changed almost beyond recognition and since 1982 general managers have usurped the lords of the manor.

What Next?

After over 30 years working in the NHS I am convinced medical practice has changed and am equally convinced that the structure within which we deliver health care must change too. The principles of equality of access to health care for all the population, of efficiency of treatment so that resources are not squandered on avoidable complications, of effectiveness so that only proven therapies are applied and outdated practices discarded, are the only clear tenets I adhere to. Like many doctors I am unsure about the capacity of 'market forces' alone to distribute health care. Medicine needs regulation with a powerful consumer input. Quality assurance programmes and better regulation to respond to consumerism will possibly achieve higher standards quicker than unfettered market provision.

Part 2

Orthopaedic Surgery

Michael Freeman

The Author

Michael Freeman was educated at Stowe School from 1945 to 1950 and at Corpus Christi College, Cambridge, from 1950 to 1953. He was a clinical medical student at The London Hospital for the following three years, qualifying MB, BCH at Cambridge in 1956. Thereafter he worked at The London Hospital, Westminster Hospital and the Middlesex Hospital before returning to his present post as Consultant Orthopaedic Surgeon at The London Hospital in 1968. He became a Fellow of the Royal College of Surgeons of England in 1959 and obtained his MD at Cambridge in 1964.

Mr Freeman has part-authored several books on orthopaedic surgery and allied subjects and published a variety of papers on orthopaedic surgery and biomechanics. He is a past President of the International Hip Society and the current President of the British Hip Society.

2

Orthopaedic Surgery

Orthopaedic surgery deals with elective (i.e. non-urgent) procedures to bones and joints. The counterpart of this specialty in the emergency field deals with the management of fractures and joint injuries. The specialty dates back to the late 19th and early 20th century when it was principally concerned with the management of bone and joint tuberculosis, poliomyelitis and a variety of congenital deformities. At that time the number of operative surgical procedures that could be performed for these conditions was limited, and much of the treatment offered took the form of braces and prolonged periods of splintage and bed rest.

Over the years the nature of orthopaedic surgery has changed totally. The introduction of antibiotics and improved hygiene has led to the virtual disappearance of bone and joint tuberculosis. Acute infection of bone, a condition which used to be relatively common and often fatal in children, has almost disappeared for reasons that are not entirely clear but which owe something to improved living conditions and (in terms of treatment as against prevention) to the use of antibiotics. Poliomyelitis has disappeared in the West with the introduction of vaccination. Many congenital deformities, for example congenital dislocation of the hip and congenital club foot, can now be detected at birth before subsequent growth has allowed important structural abnormalities to develop in the skeleton. As a consequence, they can be treated in such a way as to leave the adult patient essentially normal. Thus the procedures which formed the bulk if not the whole of an orthopaedic surgeon's activity in the 1920s have largely disappeared. Had they not been replaced with other activities, the specialty itself would also have disappeared.

Growth of this Specialty

In fact the specialty, far from contracting, has grown because of the introduction of a variety of surgical procedures for arthritis. The term 'arthritis' is used here in the broad sense to include any abnormality, be it inflammatory or degenerative, in any of the joints in the body including the spine. In practice these conditions fall into two categories. On the one hand there are the inflammatory arthropathies, the cause of which is not clearly understood and of which the principal representative is rheumatoid arthritis. This condition for reasons which are unknown is more prevalent in some communities than others, the United Kingdom being one of those in which it is relatively common. The incidence of rheumatoid arthritis in the population as a whole is thought to be approximately 1-2 per cent.

On the other hand there is a group of conditions known as 'osteoarthrosis' which affects any joint and which may be precipitated by some mechanical or structural abnormality (e.g. that produced by a previous fracture or abnormality of development) or which occurs simply with ageing. Since the expectation of life in all developed countries is increasing, the number of patients developing degenerative joint disease of symptomatic significance is also increasing. The commonest locations for osteoarthritis to make itself symptomatically manifest are the hip, knee and spine. Since much back pain is in fact of unknown causation and not clearly due to degenerative changes in the intervertebral discs or joints of the spine, the hip and knee are the most commonly involved in terms of pain and disability caused by osteoarthritis.

It will be obvious that although disabling, pain and stiffness in, say, one hip cannot in any way shorten a patient's life. Thus none of the surgery offered for patients with these conditions is 'essential' in the sense of life-saving. This contrasts with the surgery undertaken by orthopaedic surgeons of the past to treat, for example, acute osteomyelitis or tuberculosis.

It will also be obvious that in a society in which the expectation of life is little more than 40 or 50 years, degenerative joint disease represents an entirely negligible clinical problem. Orthopaedic surgeons are thus confronted with a need to consider surgery in patients who are living longer as a consequence of other improvements in medical care, and perhaps particularly as a consequence of improvement in the general standard of life, but who as they age become disabled and thus suffer a loss in the quality of their life. The arguments for operating on patients in this clinical category range from very weak to very strong. Rarely is surgery impossible and rarely is it imperative. This range of necessity is best illustrated by example.

Examples

To take a first example, strictly speaking from the field of trauma rather than that of the arthritides, consider an elderly lady who suffers a fracture of the upper end of the thigh bone adjacent to the hip. This fracture is extremely common and is caused by the thinning of the bones as the skeleton ages. In the past, this fracture used to be treated by the application of a plaster cast, and a frequent outcome was death as a consequence of inactivity and pneumonia.   Today certain of these fractures can be treated by fixing the fracture fragments together at operation with the hope that they will unite. In others however it is obvious that union cannot be expected because of the displacement at the fracture site. The upper end of the thigh bone is therefore replaced. If this is done successfully, the patient will return to a relatively normal life, walking, being comfortable and independent. Obviously many of these patients are frail or have other illnesses (for example heart failure or diabetes) at the time when they break their hip. For them the risks of surgery are considerable. It is not always possible to arrange for highly experienced anaesthetists and surgeons to be available to do these operations (at any rate in the United Kingdom) because of a shortage of orthopaedic surgeons in the population as a whole. Even if optimal anaesthesia and orthopaedic surgery were available, some of these patients might not survive an operation. Equally they would not survive were they to be untreated, since to be confined to bed in the clinical conditions visualised almost always results in hypostatic pneumonia and death. Thus all such patients are in practice operated on and although the operation is not strictly life-saving, its impact on the quality of life and the expectation of life is such as to make it universally agreed that some form of operative procedure is required.

Consider now a somewhat different fracture, involving the socket of the hip joint, which has united but in an anatomically imperfect way. As a consequence over the next five years the hip develops degenerative changes so that now the patient notices that he is unable to walk for, say, more than 15 minutes because of pain, that pain in the hip disturbs his sleep and that stiffness makes it impossible for him to reach his foot to put on his shoe. Theoretically this situation could again be treated by hip replacement or by an operation known as arthrodesis in which pain is abolished but at the price of totally stiffening the hip joint.

If the patient is 85 and in poor health it might be thought better to advise acceptance of the disability rather than to run the risks of operative surgery which at that age might end in death. If the patient is 65, the quality of life compared with what it would be if the hip were essentially normal is so gravely impaired that most patients will accept hip replacement as a solution to their problem: hip replacement if successful (and 95 per cent of such operations are) will effectively abolish pain, enable the patient to walk and to reach his foot: in short to lead a normal life for a man of 65.

If the patient is 25 the issue alters again. Now hip replacement is certain not to last the patient's lifetime and if it fails will leave her grossly disabled. Most surgeons in these circumstances would offer the patient the stiffening operation since although this will not abolish the disability it will get rid of pain and will last a lifetime. A woman aged 25 may still prefer to accept pain if she has movement at the hip rather than have the hip permanently stiffened or to have it replaced leaving her to face even greater disability in her thirties. Thus exactly the same clinical condition represents a clear-cut argument for surgery at the age of 65, a questionable argument for surgery at the age of 25 and possibly no argument for surgery at the age of 85.

The Impact of Aging

Far more common than degenerative changes brought about by a fracture are degenerative changes in the hip brought about simply by the passage of time. This condition becomes increasingly common after the age of 60 although it can occasionally develop for no evident precipitating reason at younger ages. The patient may first notice a little aching discomfort in the hip after he has walked for an hour or two, say playing 18 holes of golf. Later the hip may become slightly stiff but not sufficiently so to disturb any day-to-day activity. Eventually sleep may be disturbed on an occasional night. As the condition increases, the length of time the patient can be on his feet before pain becomes intolerable shortens and may eventually get to the point at which walking is hardly possible. Sleep is disturbed. Stiffness of the hip (which is accompanied by a cross-legged deformity) may become so severe as to make it impossible to carry out normal toilet activities. Since the condition can affect both hips it led, in elderly patients before surgery was a possibility, to a condition in which the patient was bed bound with the legs fixed permanently in a cross-legged position and in permanent pain. Many patients would regard death as preferable. In an initial effort to reduce this final disability an operation was devised early in this century in which the thigh bone was broken and reset so as at least to correct the deformity and reduce the disability from the toilet point of view.

Surprisingly this was sometimes found to relieve pain and was therefore used as a pain-relieving procedure for many years. Now however the operation of hip replacement, introduced by two English surgeons, McKee and Charnley in the 1960s, has revolutionised the management of this disease: a successful hip replacement can produce a joint which, in the context of the lifestyle of a man of 65, can be indistinguishable from normal. The question arises: at what stage in the development of an osteoarthrosic hip should hip replacement be considered? The surgeon's responsibility here is neither to refuse surgery nor to impose it. Rather he should explain to the patient what might be the hazards of the operation: it can for example fail because of some anaesthetic catastrophe, because the implant comes loose in later years, or because the joint becomes infected. Any of these things may leave the patient worse for surgical intervention, not better. The surgeon must explain what lifestyle can be expected without treatment or after a successful operation. He must give an estimation of the chances, in his hands, of achieving a successful outcome. It must then be left for the patient to decide whether his disability is severe enough to merit the unpleasantness and risks of surgery. Roughly speaking if a patient is 65 or over and has a significant disturbance of sleep accompanied by an inability to walk for 30 minutes, it is unusual for a patient to elect to accept disability rather than to be operated on. At the other extreme, a man of 50 who, because he is younger, is more likely eventually to suffer the complication of a loose implant and who at the time of presenting to the doctor has no greater disability than that he cannot play 18 holes of golf may not accept surgery and would be wise to take this decision. There is therefore no absolute moment at which surgery becomes indicated for this disease: it is a question of the patient's age, expectation of life, expectation of lifestyle in his remaining years, general health and tolerance for pain.

Degenerative Joint Disease in the Knee

The situation at the knee is very similar to that of the hip. Early in the onset of degenerative joint disease in the knee, a patient may have little disability other than that he cannot engage in his accustomed sports. In the United Kingdom this would generally speaking not be regarded as an appropriate indication for surgery. However in the USA the cultural attitudes of both patient and surgeon alike would make this a disability that many elderly retired people would have difficulty accepting. They might therefore prefer to have their knee operated upon rather than give up golf. One can only speculate as to how this difference comes about. Partly it is connected with the greater number of orthopaedic surgeons per head of population in the USA as against the United Kingdom and partly, perhaps, because there is a widespread attitude in the United States that disability and illness are in a sense signs of inadequacy and defeat. Thus it is not socially acceptable to accept one's disability rather than to try and 'conquer' it.

As degenerative changes in the knee progress they commonly come to affect both legs. Now the disability becomes of greater significance although pain at night, in contrast to the situation at the hip, is often absent until late in the disease thus at least making it possible for the patient to sleep. However, significant degenerative changes in both knees will materially reduce the distance a patient can walk and in particular interferes with their use of stairs. Like degenerative change in the hip, this threatens the independence of an elderly person for whom no prospect may be worse than that of having to give up their homes because they can no longer manage physically. Thus many patients will elect to have their knee replaced if both sides are involved and the disability has reached the level described.

The question then arises: should one knee be operated on or both? If only one is replaced the patient's disability is often not greatly improved since the other knee remains as a significant handicap. If both knees are replaced the patient has to contemplate two significant operations separated by a period of rehabilitation between the two, a total treatment programme which can be daunting. Today it is common, in centres carrying out knee replacement in significant numbers and where therefore the surgeons are sufficiently experienced, for both knees to be replaced under one anaesthetic. This raises a further variable in the spectrum of treatment choices, namely the experience of the surgeon and anaesthetist whom the patient consults. An experienced knee replacement surgeon working with a good anaesthetist will not hesitate today to replace both knees. An inexperienced surgeon may elect not to replace either knee simply because he is unsure of the outcome of this operation in his hands.

Thus not only is the decision to operate influenced by the patient's disability and his attitude to that disability, his social setting, and his general health, it is also influenced by the experience of the doctors to whom he goes for treatment.

Rheumatoid Arthritis

Finally it is appropriate to consider the situation confronting patients with rheumatoid arthritis. Many of these patients are young adults, often women. More than one joint is involved. A woman may marry and start a family before developing the disease. In her late twenties she may develop rheumatoid changes which affect first one knee then the other, and then perhaps one hip, each joint causing a significant disability. Such a woman is confronted with the breakdown of her marriage and an inability not only to care for herself but (a disability often more important to a mother), an inability to care for her children. Because joint replacement cannot be guaranteed to last the lifetime of someone of this age, the surgeon will ordinarily hesitate to consider replacing the knee in a patient in their thirties: a woman with mild pain in her knee would certainly not be considered for this procedure. On the other hand there is no alternative to joint replacement for the mother in the example now being considered than a wheelchair.

Many women will say that they would be happy to face whatever the long-term future may bring, including a wheelchair, if only they can be rendered able-bodied during the childhood and adolescence of their children. This means that the knee would be replaced in a woman of 30. If rheumatoid changes continue a second knee will be replaced followed perhaps by a hip. These procedures may then fail when the patient is in her forties, requiring revision operations which are technically difficult and demanding of resources. Eventually revision may be impractical and the patient will require a wheelchair.

From the point of view of resource management it could perhaps be argued that it would have been just as appropriate to have arranged a wheelchair at the outset as to subject the woman in this example to a series of expensive procedures eventually ending in the same outcome. From the patient's point of view however, with her children in mind, there is absolutely no question as to which is preferable. One thus has to bear in mind not only the impact on the patient, not only the skills and attitude of the surgeon, not only the attitudes of society, but also the attitudes and interests of the family.

A Matter of Judgement

It may be concluded that the arguments for or against surgery throughout this area of medicine are almost entirely a matter of judgement. There are no absolute indications either for operating or for refraining from operating. In the past societies have prospered in the total absence of procedures of this kind.

Today some societies (the USA for example) employ joint replacement procedures more frequently than others (such as the UK) with no obvious reason for the discrepancy. Ultimately the surgeon's role is to explain to the patient what the pros and cons of surgery as opposed to acceptance of the disability might be. Clearly the surgeon must make a decision as to whether or not the patient is a responsible individual who can then make a decision for himself, and he must ask whether the disability seems severe enough to make replacement surgery, broadly speaking, appropriate. Once that is done the patient, who is in the last analysis the only person who experiences both the disability and the procedure, must make up his own mind. In doing that patients are naturally influenced by the cultural milieu in which they live; specifically they will be influenced by the opinions and experiences of their acquaintances who may have had similar surgery.

Economic Factors

Since reconstructive procedures on arthritic joints now represent a substantial proportion of elective surgery in the UK, the conclusion that the whole of the field is subject to matters of personal judgement rather than absolute indications for surgery has considerable implications for overall medical expenditure.

The relative nature of the medical indications for an operation such as knee replacement can be illustrated by reference to the effect of economic and cultural factors.

From the economic point of view, consider three Polish patients. The first, who remained in his native Poland, would not be able to get his knee replaced under any circumstances: the prosthesis is too expensive for the medical services to purchase and as a consequence the operation is unknown. If such a patient's knee became intolerably painful he would either have to use a wheelchair if that were available or have his knee surgically stiffened. At the other extreme imagine a patient who emigrated from Poland to America and retired to Florida where there is approximately one orthopaedic surgeon to 15,000 of population. At this level, orthopaedic surgeons are looking for work and the Polish patient now might be advised to have his knee replaced simply because pain interfered with 18 holes of golf. Between these two extremes, consider a patient who emigrated to England where there are 1.39 consultant orthopaedic surgeons per 100,000 population. At that level of orthopaedic provision, waiting lists for elective orthopaedic surgery are universal and only significantly disabled patients have their knee replaced. Thus, a man in England might get his knee replaced if he was unable to walk for 20 minutes, but would be advised to change his recreations if pain interfered with golf.

Cultural Factors

From the cultural point of view, consider the effect of knee replacement upon the amount that the knee will bend. Roughly speaking, after knee replacement the knee will flex through about 100 degrees going from fully straight to bent rather more than a right angle. The normal knee will of course flex more than this until the heel touches the buttock.

In the West, flexion beyond 100 degrees is not essential and patients therefore will readily accept this loss of movement if in return they lose the pain. In Japan however, it is culturally imperative for women to be able to kneel seated on their heels. A Japanese woman might therefore be very reluctant to have her knee replaced however painful it was.

In India the poor squat, again sitting on their heels. Knee replacement is not available for the poor of India but if it were to be, the patients would be severely incapacitated after operation unless they had chairs in their houses.

In some sheikdoms of the Middle East, it is imperative to be seated on the floor in the presence of the ruler. This may be difficult if neither knee flexes beyond 90 degrees. If one cannot be seated in the presence of the ruler, one cannot have access to the ruler — a major cultural disadvantage for many patients in such a country. Thus knee replacement would be accepted by patients with great reluctance, if at all.

Part 3

Doctors Making Decisions

James Le Fanu

The Author

James Le Fanu is a Medical Columnist on *The Independent on Sunday* and a General Practitioner in South London. A graduate of Cambridge and The London Hospital he has taken a special interest in studying the patterns of disease.

Dr Le Fanu is the author of *Eat Your Heart Out - The Fallacy of a Health Diet* (London, MacMillan, 1987) and is currently working on a health guide for the over sixties. He is Medical Advisor to the independent television company Meditel.

3

Doctors Making Decisions

A major plank of the Government's offensive in favour of its NHS reforms *Working for Patients*[1] are the statistics generated by the Department of Health showing major variations between districts in prescribing and referral policies, waiting lists and so on. The assumption is that there are a series of causes to explain these variations, which were they identified and modified in favour of greater efficiency would resolve most of the problems of the NHS. If, however, the major contributory factors to these variations are not structural but rather arise from philosophical and temperamental differences in decision making by doctors, then it is likely to be much more difficult to achieve the desired aim of raising standards throughout the country to the level of the most efficient and cost effective.

The question of what does indeed influence a doctor's decision in favour of one course of clinical management as opposed to another has received scant attention in the literature and I will attempt to illustrate it with a recent case history.

A Case Study

A 67-year-old retired labourer, whom I knew quite well as a phlegmatic, albeit not very bright, old codger, came to the surgery one day to tell me that when he walked down the street he felt as if he, 'had had a few too many — I'm pitching around like a ship in a storm'.

---

[1] *Working for Patients*, Cm 555, London: HMSO, January 1989.

Examining him confirmed what I had suspected — that there was something awry with the cerebellar part of the brain which controls co-ordination. In view of his age and the acute onset of symptoms this was probably vascular in origin, i.e. he had had a small stroke. His blood pressure was normal, so I gave him a prescription for aspirin, advised him his symptoms would improve over the next two weeks and made a further appointment to see him. When he returned he had indeed improved, and was fully recovered within another month.

Other doctors would, no doubt, have managed this case differently. Following the case history and examination the patient would have had a few haematological and biochemical tests to 'exclude' potentially exacerbating causes of his symptoms like anaemia or diabetes. He would have had a chest X-ray because sometimes carcinoma of the bronchus can present in this manner, either as a secondary lesion or as a paraneoplastic syndrome. He would have had an ECG to exclude a recent myocardial infarct which can occasionally result in thrombus formation and a scattering of blood clots to the brain, and an echocardiagram to examine the shape and configuration of the heart muscle. He might have had a 24-hour tape as, occasionally, intermittent cardiac conduction abnormalities can result in a sudden fall of blood pressure leading to a stroke. He would have had an X-ray of the cervical spine as occasionally cervical spondylitis can lead to pressure on the vertebro-basilar arteries that feed the cerebellum.

If the results of all these investigations were normal then he would have been referred to a neurologist where parts of this process would be repeated and he would then have a MRI scan, which is the best way of visualising lesions in the cerebellum and could either confirm the diagnosis or exclude other possible causes such as neoplasm (primary or secondary), or a demyelinating disease like multiple sclerosis. Were it to confirm the original diagnosis of a stroke he would undergo digital subtraction angiography (DSA) to visualise the cerebrovascular arterial tree lest there be a stenotic lesion that might be amenable to surgery. At the end of all this he would be prescribed aspirin, and advised his symptoms were likely to improve.

The differences in management policy of this one patient, even though the outcome is the same, is hardly worth emphasising. The financial cost of the first approach is virtually zero. With the second, if one counts in the amount of doctors' time as well as all the investigations, there is unlikely to be much change from £5,000. The cost to the patient of the first approach is again virtually nil as he had been fully reassured that he will recover. The same cannot be said for the second approach, where the physical discomfort and time spent undergoing the many investigations, the anxiety and uncertainty that they invariably generate might all be considered an unwelcome and unnecessary burden on the patient.

Using this case as an example, it is possible to tease out the many, varied influences on how doctors reach decisions.

Knowledge and Experience

It is easy to see how a general practitioner who had taken a special interest in neurological problems during his training, or indeed had done a neurological job as part of a vocational training scheme, would react to this case but probably only a minority of GPs confronted by this story and after physical examination could confidently make a diagnosis of a vascular mid-line cerebellar lesion, though in truth they certainly should be capable of doing so. Many therefore might opt to refer initially for a specialist opinion, with all the financial and psychological implications this would entail. The point here is that the level of competence is an immensely powerful influence on GPs' decision making. When general practice encompasses, as it does, the full range of abilities from Cambridge graduates with starred firsts in their thirties to moribund old characters in their seventies, then it seems almost impossible to generalise about the type and quality of decisions that are made by GPs.

But even if the doctor were able to make the diagnosis with a fair degree of certainty, this still allows for the two extremes of management outlined: either no investigation and firm reassurance, or the view that this is 'an interesting case' which should be 'worked up' with a view to excluding possible rare remediable causes. A possible compromise that would link the two management philosophies would be to allow the 'time factor' to operate. Here it would be decided that on a basis of probabilities this is likely to be a vascular lesion that will improve spontaneously, and so the initial plan would be to observe. If, however, there is no sign of improvement after two weeks this might be the time to initiate further investigations.

'Philosophical Differences'

Nonetheless GPs with similar experience do pursue very different management policies, and here I think the fundamental difference is 'philosophical', that is doctors' different philosophies of medicine. This can be summarised as the position they take on the gradient between minimalism and interventionism.

Putting it simply, if the only interest is the welfare of the patient, then one would choose the management plan that would reduce to a minimum the treadmill of investigation and treatment. If, however, the real fascination is with medicine itself, the utilisation of the wide range of investigations that are available, the pursuit of the clever but rare diagnosis, then one is obviously much more likely to fall into the interventionist camp. There are, of course, a whole host of other influences on where one stands on the minimalist — interventionist axis. The busy doctor is less likely to be interventionist, the old doctor is more likely to be sanguine about the wonders of modern medicine, boredom and disillusionment encourage a more nihilistic attitude, and so on.

The tension between minimalism and interventionism is readily seen in the notes of any patient who is under the care of a large group practice. The younger, junior partners may record half a page of notes on the most trivial symptoms, while their middle-aged senior partner who has long since lost any interest other than in the scale of fees will record an illegible few words of scrawl.

The Doctor/Patient Relationship

The patient has a powerful influence on the way in which doctors make their decisions, so, turning to the original example, I am sure that if the patient in question had been under the doctor for many years, consulted him successfully on previous occasions and trusted him accordingly, and if this was reciprocated then the patient would have the confidence to accept that his symptoms, though obviously serious, could none the less be quite adequately managed by his general practitioner.

But it is easy to imagine how this might not be the case. A nervous patient might merit further investigation, if only for reassurance (it is remarkable how frequently patients with headaches which often stretch back many years now request a brain scan to make sure they do not have a tumour).

The middle-class patient would be expected to have a better idea of what the differential diagnosis might be, and what medicine can offer in the way of investigation and would expect a bit more than a pat on the back and firm reassurance. But it is also to do with expectations; the middle class, often taking a generally disdainful view of general practice, would in these circumstances expect a specialist opinion.

As one would anticipate, medico-legal considerations play an important role in decision making in the United States. The highly unlikely probability of there being a very rare cause of the presenting syndrome does not convince an American Court of Law that the doctor should not have diligently done all in his powers to exclude it.

A subtler but related phenomenon in Britain is the possibility of litigation from relatives especially if, for example, there was a fatal outcome. So even if the GP was confident the diagnosis was a small cerebellar stroke that would improve spontaneously, the possibility remains that the patient might have a further episode which could be catastrophic even though nothing could be done to prevent it. The relatives might well see things differently, noting that the patient had been to see the doctor, say four weeks previously, that the doctor had appeared to do nothing and had not even bothered to refer the patient to hospital for further attention. Unaware of the subtleties of the case and how the GP was endeavouring to spare the patient unnecessary investigation, along with the need for relatives to assuage their guilt that they themselves should have done more, the GP's approach could easily be interpreted as negligence. The prospect of aggravation from relatives in circumstances such as this is an important factor in opting for hospital referral.

Finally, there is the crucial question of the personality of patients. Early on in general practice I became aware of the 'thin folder' syndrome. In this patients, perhaps in their sixties or seventies, come to the surgery, their notes only comprise one or two cards and it is apparent that the last time they consulted was a decade or so ago. Immediately the antennae of clinical suspicion are raised. These patients have to be listened to very carefully and the symptoms they describe taken seriously indeed. The likelihood is that they are only 'bothering the doctor' because there is something seriously wrong for which they need help. The other extreme, the 'thick folder' syndrome, describes patients in their mid twenties whose folders can be twenty times as thick and includes a sheaf of hospital letters from a galaxy of consultants which reveal that little, if anything, has ever been found to be seriously the matter.

Why has this patient received so much medical attention? The GP may have been mystified by her symptoms, unable to help her, anxious to get her off his back and so given in to pressure for a specialist opinion. Here we see how frequently decision making in practice has relatively little to do with objective needs shrewdly assessed, but rather is determined by the wider problem of how to manage patients whom neurosis or hypochondriasis has turned into chronic attenders.

Health Service Organisation

This paper opened by observing the current political significance of the question of how GPs make decisions. The issue is whether the mode of organisation of health services is sufficiently influential to override the major determinants of decision making already considered and which might be thought essentially unmodifiable: the personality of doctor and patient, their attitude to and expectations from medicine.

(a) *Private Medicine*

Private general practice is rare in Britain, presumably because at this level the NHS provides a service that most find satisfactory. To stay in business the private GP must provide a personalised service, give the patients more time than they would get in the National Health Service, and in more congenial surroundings. One presumes that most of those who do have a private general practitioner are not unduly concerned about cost.

These features combined tend to influence medical decision making in favour of over-investigation and over- treatment. In the example of the man in his sixties, the perceived value of private medicine, that is the quality of service, makes it likely that the exhaustive investigations suggested, with subsequent specialist referral would be almost inevitable. There is a further incentive to investigate if the doctor either runs his own laboratory, has his own X-ray facilities or is involved in a network of mutual referrals whereby spreading his patients' money around his colleagues would be rewarded either by boosting his own reputation, or getting referrals from other doctors.

Similar factors operate when dealing with more trivial conditions. When remuneration is dependent not only on how many patients one has, but also how often they are seen, there is a natural tendency routinely to follow up problems at regular intervals, to institute treatment where a policy of procrastination would be more appropriate, and to investigate a possible organic basis for symptoms which are quite clearly neurotic.

(b) *The NHS*

Few, if any, of these influences operate in the National Health Service: if anything the reverse is the case. Under the new proposed contract for general practitioners where remuneration is based on number of patients, there is likely to be an incentive to minimise the number and frequency of follow-up appointments lest the surgery get too crowded or waiting list for appointments become too long. On the other hand, with open-ended budgets, and easy referral there is little imperative to think vigorously about what might be the best — the most appropriate and cost-effective, method of dealing with medical problems when they occur.

(c) *Budget holding practices*

It is only possible to speculate on how the introduction of budget holding in general practice might improve decision making to overcome the disadvantages of private or NHS-style medicine.

Health maintenance organisations provide a clue, with their diagnostic related groups in which standard forms of investigation and treatment are laid down for defined conditions. Here decisions about management are taken out of the hands of doctors in the name of established policy and there is no doubt that this could overcome the vagaries of decision making arising from, for example, an individual doctor's attitude to medicine, or a patient's expectation.

It must be stressed however that the scope here is limited almost exclusively to quite clear-cut clinical situations invariably involving elective surgery.

But one could imagine that the experience of being in a budget-holding practice might allow doctors to generalise from that experience to think more vigorously about how they are managing a wider set of clinical conditions. Again, invoking our original example, this might tilt the balance in favour of a conservative expectant approach to the management of cerebellar strokes as opposed to an interventionist investigatory one.

In summary then, one case history of a man in his sixties with a cerebellar stroke illustrates the enormous spectrum of influences on the ways doctors approach clinical problems.

In reality medical practice is probably less anarchic than this account suggests. Though it is difficult to generalise, most doctors seem to operate what is best described as 'an internal audit'. Medical problems found in general practice are rarely complex and fall into a few broad categories and after a time in practice doctors learn instinctively what needs to be done in a way that cannot be taught and is not readily amenable to analysis. Thus 'internal audit' is a subconscious or subliminal phenomenon bolstered by shared training and assumptions and a shared professional ethic that ensures doctors will, to a large extent, share a commonality of outlook in dealing with clinical problems. It balances the needs of the patient for a proper diagnosis and the most up to date and effective treatment against the blind application of technology to medical problems.

Yet I have suggested that the diversity of medical decision making can be explained at least in part in terms of doctors' temperaments and patients' attitudes, and it is equally true that conflicts about what exactly is the right thing to do are always present in the practice of a single doctor. So to conclude I have taken one of my surgeries at random to show how even with the internal audit working at full tilt, the dilemmas focused by clinical problems raise considerable uncertainties as to what indeed is the right decision in any single case.

Case 1: *A 36-year-old male with fungal infection of the scrotum.*

The infection is easily treated with appropriate medication but as the patient had not had his blood pressure previously recorded, the opportunity was taken to do so, and it was 150 over 100. Fifteen years ago this would have merited hospital referral with extensive investigations including catecholamine measurements and intravenous urography to exclude a remediable underlying cause but the very low yield of a positive diagnosis has meant this approach has subsequently fallen into disrepute. It is now more likely that he will be recalled on several occasions over the next three or four months for further blood pressure estimations and this is what I intend to do. However, even if the blood pressure remained elevated the question of whether treatment at this level is beneficial remains very unclear. There is some small benefit in terms of reducing strokes from treating mild hypertension, but the cost in terms of drugs taken, possible side effects, the neuroticism associated with a diagnosis of 'high blood pressure' is difficult to calculate. As a minimalist I would probably opt for nothing and merely observe him over the next few years, but I recognise that many other doctors would dispute this decision.

Case 2: *An 83-year-old man with fixed angina pectoris unable to walk more than 50 yards, despite being on optimal medical treatment.*

There is nothing more that a GP has to offer this man and the next logical step is for him to be referred to hospital for further investigation and the consideration of coronary angioplasty. The likelihood, however, of finding a lesion that is amenable to this type of approach and which would be beneficial must be very small indeed. As I know the patient quite well I feel the appropriate course, rather than raising false hopes, is to attempt to reconcile this patient to his disability. However, it is quite easy to imagine that were the patient to find it difficult to accept this advice, or were there pressure from other sources such as relatives, then one would have no alternative other than to seek a specialist opinion.

Case 3: *A 19-year-old with moderate acne.*

This young man has had acne for five years which is controlled, though not completely, with regular antibiotic medication. He has recently heard of a new drug, Retin A, and he has come with a request for a prescription. His case is not severe enough to warrant this treatment though it is likely to be more effective than what he is currently taking. Here we are dealing with a patient with a very low threshold for the inconvenience and embarrassment of an aesthetic problem. This might be in itself a reason to give in to his pressure, but it is difficult to justify on clearly clinical grounds.

Case 4: *A 45-year-old woman with a long history of anxiety and somatic symptoms, requests a repeat prescription of the tranquillizer Lorazepam.*

There is now widespread hostility amongst doctors to the repeat prescription of benzodiazepine tranquillizers and another doctor might well make a repeat prescription conditional on a plan of phased withdrawal with associated psychotherapy. I have never found this, personally, a successful approach, and as time has passed, have become convinced that just as diabetics need insulin there is a small group of patients who require regular anti-anxiolytic medication.

Case 5: *A 76-year-old woman comes with her daughter complaining of being 'off her feet', and with left upper chest pain.*

I have already seen this woman on one occasion when her physical examination was essentially normal. I reassured her on that occasion but this time, with pressure from relatives, I agreed to some baseline investigations including a chest X-ray and an ECG. These subsequently turned out to be essentially normal though the chest X-ray showed some enlargement of the heart. Three days after this consultation I was told this patient was found dead at home by her son. In retrospect the symptoms she described were those of a pre-morbid state, which without being able to put one's finger on exactly what is wrong, invariably ends with a fatal outcome. Though I am sure that nothing I could have done for this woman would have been beneficial, I could sympathise with her relatives, who are also my patients, if they were to think that I had not done enough for her when she initially came for consultation.

Case 6: *A 36-year-old man with gout.*

This man had an acute episode of gout ten days previously and had improved with anti-inflammatory medication. However, his uric acid measurement was only in the upper limits of normal so though I do not doubt the clinical diagnosis, the question now is whether he should be placed on long-term anti-gout medication to prevent a further flare up in future. There is a small probability that patients not so treated end with chronic renal failure. An option here would be to keep the patient under review and measure his uric acid levels perhaps yearly. However, as the likelihood is that he would fail to attend for follow-up appointments, it might therefore be easiest to start him on the appropriate drugs now.

Case 7: *A 47-year-old woman with menopausal symptoms, taking hormone replacement therapy on which she is much improved.*

Routine measurement of blood pressure reveals that she is mildly hypertensive on this occasion, which is a theoretical contra-indication to the continuation of HRT. Were she to have a stroke in the next two or three years, even though it might not be related to her current treatment, the failure to have discontinued it might well be considered grounds for negligence at some future date. On the other hand she is so debilitated by her menopausal symptoms and has improved so dramatically with the HRT it seems kindest to continue therapy.

Case 8: *A 72-year-old man with a history of weight loss.*

This man who had gastrectomy in the past complains of anorexia and weight loss of a stone and a half over the previous two months. I have extensively investigated him for possible metabolic or neoplastic cause of his symptoms and have turned up nothing. It now seems that the probable cause of his symptoms might be a depressive illness. However, hospital referral would seem to be obligatory even though I am sceptical the hospital specialist would finding anything that I have missed.

Case 9: *A 27-year-old woman with 'post-viral syndrome'.*

I have been taken for a ride by this patient who initially presented with symptoms of a viral illness, subsequently complained that she was weak and unable to concentrate, and later informed me that she was suffering from post-viral syndrome, or ME. I have done a multiplicity of investigations and given her extensive time off work to aid recovery. In a sense I have colluded with the patient's diagnosis and it is now difficult to extricate myself. She is now convinced that her symptoms are dietary in origin and requests a referral to an allergy specialist at a London teaching hospital. If I want an easy life then it seems sensible to spend a couple of minutes writing the referral letter. If I confront her with the probable diagnosis of hysterical manipulation, I will almost certainly get nowhere. I decided to write the referral letter.

Case 10: *A 29-year-old man with psoriasis.*

This man's mild psoriasis has been adequately controlled with cold tar and steroid preparations. He now wishes a referral to a dermatologist because he maintains he is sure there is something more that can be done. I am sure that there is not, but when he says he wishes to go privately I raise no objections.

Case 11: *A 55-year-old woman with arthritis.*

This patient has arthritis confined to one joint and has no previous symptoms. There is a possibility that this could be the first sign of a more generalised and serious arthritic illness such as rheumatoid but in my experience most cases of mono-arthritis settle spontaneously and there are no further sequelae. Were I more fascinated by the spectrum of arthritic illness, I would certainly suggest a series of investigations to identify an underlying cause or the possibility of a more serious illness. Instead I took her full blood count and ESR which will cost the NHS about 5p. I advised local treatment along with some anti-inflammatory drugs and arranged to see her the next week.

Dilemmas of Clinical Management

Each of these cases presented dilemmas of clinical management with considerable cost implications. The advantage of working within the National Health Service, in its present form, is that any decision that is reached can be fairly assumed to be based on an evaluation of the pros and cons of different management options. The introduction of budget-holding would appear to favour a conservative, non-interventionist approach to medical practice which is what I strive for myself.

The difference is between such an approach which is freely arrived at, and one which is required by external constraints, such as the need to remain within one's budget.

Part 4

One Tuesday Afternoon

Brian S. Mantell

The Author

Brian Mantell MRCP, FRCR, qualified from The London Hospital Medical College, University of London, in 1958. Since 1970, he has been Consultant in Radiotherapy and Oncology to The London Hospital and The National Heart and Chest Hospitals. He is Honorary Senior Lecturer at The National Heart and Lung Institute and Honorary Consultant in Radiotherapy and Oncology to East Roding Hospitals.

Dr Mantell is married to a Consultant Physician in Genito-Urinary Medicine and has two children. He lives in Dulwich, South London.

4

One Tuesday Afternoon

It was Tuesday lunch time when the consultant radiotherapist and oncologist arrived at the district hospital for his fortnightly peripheral clinic. It was a fine bright day, traffic had been light, and he welcomed the change of scene from the regional cancer centre at the university hospital in the city, 30 miles away. At lunch he met the senior surgeon, one of whose patients he was to see in his clinic. This was, the surgeon told him, an intelligent and attractive woman of 35, who had found a lump in the right breast, perhaps half an inch in diameter. Mammography followed by a needle aspiration had confirmed that it was a carcinoma. The patient led a busy life; in addition to caring for her family, she worked part-time as a journalist for the local newspaper.

The First Patient

Twenty minutes later the two doctors met the patient. She was well aware that she had breast cancer and that investigations had shown no evidence of spread to her liver or skeleton; she did not know of the doctors' unease that in spite of the negative investigations such spread might indeed be present and could declare itself months or years later. Should they tell her that? Would it help the three of them to decide on treatment? Or would it merely add to her anxiety to no useful end?

The surgeon remembered that when he was learning his craft the treatment for such a case was well known — radical mastectomy was required as soon as possible to remove the breast and its draining glands before the cancer was able to spread, as it was believed. But this had long been shown to be a false supposition — cure is not influenced by the extent of the surgery. Nowadays such patients preferred to be treated by removal of only part of the breast — avoiding mutilating surgery and preserving the patient's feminine image of herself. With the addition of post-operative radiotherapy to reduce the risk of recurrence within the breast, survival was as good as with radical mastectomy. This, therefore, was the treatment they were prepared to offer the patient. But what of the glands in the armpit which drained the breast? Should they be treated with radiotherapy? Or would it be better to remove the glands from the armpit by a surgical dissection? This would avoid the need to give radiotherapy to the armpit, giving it to the breast alone. Furthermore, it would be possible for the pathologist to say whether the glands were involved by cancer. And if they were?

The patient was well aware, as were her doctors, that in many centres involvement of the armpit glands by cancer meant that chemotherapy would be advised as there was evidence that this might prolong the time before the cancer appeared again and might possibly delay death from cancer. But chemotherapy could be unpleasant, as well as expensive and risky, and in spite of the claims of its protagonists for its benefits, it did not cure anyone, and neither surgeon nor radiotherapist advised it.

The patient however had views of her own as to how she should be treated. She felt that the breast was contaminated by cancer, and would only be happy if it were completely removed, and an implant inserted to reproduce the breast shape.

The Second Patient

The second patient had been referred from the local chest clinic. A 41-year-old area manager for a retail tobacconist chain, he had worked long and successfully in promoting his firm's profitability. A 40-a-day man himself for many years, he had regarded warnings about the dangers of cigarette smoking with scorn. But now he was ill. His face was swollen and ears blue. His collar was open to relieve the pressure of the engorged veins in which the blood was dammed up by his advanced lung cancer which was obstructing the flow to his heart. He had felt perfectly well, his normal vigorous self, until a few days previously when he had first noticed that his head felt full on bending forward. He was distressed by his illness, yet dismissed it with a certain bravado. He avoided asking his diagnosis and was anxious to return to work as soon as possible since he was looking forward to promotion to a regional post the following year, with a welcome increase in salary.

'Your patient has been referred to me from the chest clinic', wrote the radiotherapist to the family doctor. 'I shall arrange urgent palliative radiotherapy for superior vena caval obstruction caused by an anaplastic carcinoma of his right lung. His symptoms should be relieved within a few days, but I regret to say his prognosis must be very poor and I would not expect him to survive more than perhaps six months, irrespective of any treatment given.'

Other Patients

A very anxious 50-year-old postman was next. He knew he had a basal cell carcinoma on his forehead, and was convinced he faced impending death. 'Yes, this is a small skin cancer', the radiotherapist said, 'but it will not spread anywhere else. If not treated it will get bigger, but we will certainly cure it completely.' Both the radiotherapist and the surgeon were happy to treat this patient, who was offered a choice of a course of seven very quick and easy X-ray treatments, or admission as a day case for a small operation under a general anaesthetic. These two methods of treatment were thought to be equally good — which would the patient prefer? As he was unable to decide, his doctors opted for radiotherapy. There was a short waiting list of similar patients — treatment would begin in about six weeks. It was with difficulty that the patient was persuaded that this delay would not be detrimental and that his cancer would not become terminal in the interim.

One of the consultant gynaecologists had referred a 43- year-old woman. 'I shall be grateful for your advice on treatment for this patient who has a well differentiated Stage I B squamous cell carcinoma of the cervix,' he wrote. The radiotherapist had long experience of treating such patients by a combination of external and internal radiotherapy with a permanent cure rate of at least 80 per cent. But the patient herself was slim and fit and a 'good operative risk' for radical hysterectomy which produced equally good results. It might be possible to conserve her ovaries, avoiding the menopausal hot flushes which would follow radiotherapy. Which treatment should he advise? Each had its own protagonists, but no firm clinical trial gave an unequivocal answer as to which was to be preferred. Some centres routinely combined surgery and radiotherapy for such patients. Clearly the treatment given depended upon the personal preference and expertise of the specialists available rather than a firm knowledge of what was really the best.

The Patient's View

What were the patient's views? She had read an article in the popular press about a centre where chemotherapy was being added to the routine treatment allegedly with an outstanding improvement in the number of cures obtained. But this was essentially an experimental treatment, it was explained. It was expensive, unpleasant and to some extent dangerous. Its possible long-term effects were not fully understood and it was at present the subject of carefully controlled clinical trials, the results of which were still awaited. It was quite likely that no real benefit would ultimately come from such treatment and possible that harm could result. The patient remained convinced that she was being denied the chance of a certain cure that she believed had been discovered.

The radiotherapist remained with a feeling of unease that no one really knew the best treatment for this condition, given that the patient was fit for all the possible options. Which method really gives the best chance of permanent cure? Which causes fewer sequelae for the patient and the least disruption to life? How much does each cost and which is the most cost effective? 'It's the same with carcinoma of the oesophagus,' he reflected. 'There are those who believe that radical oesophagectomy, formidable a procedure as it is, gives the patient the best chance. I would rather use radical radiotherapy; that is what I would want for myself if I had that disease, but no one really knows the better option. The randomised trial comparing the two methods which I agreed to join was closed because so few patients were being entered into it. One thing I do know; once you have made the diagnosis of oesophageal carcinoma you must get on with treatment urgently, before the patient loses the ability to swallow altogether.'

Random Treatment

A man of 24 with Hodgkin's disease had returned to the clinic for a decision on treatment. The diagnosis had been made six weeks previously when an enlarged gland had been removed from his neck. The patient himself felt well. His temperature had remained normal and he had lost no weight. But the battery of investigations carried out in the interim had shown involvement of other glands — in the chest and in the abdomen. He had agreed to take part in a clinical trial, between radiotherapy to all the glands in his body, which would take about three months overall, and chemotherapy given every three weeks or so for six months. These treatments seemed to give an equal chance of permanent cure, and the trial was to determine which treatment was the better. A telephone call to the trial co-ordinator and the treatment to be given — chemotherapy — was selected at random.

The End of the Afternoon

Eighteen more patients were seen before the clinic was finished. After the clinic the radiotherapist called in at the geriatric ward where he had been requested to see a woman of 86 years. The patient was mildly confused, and had been admitted as she lived alone and was unable to care for herself. Like the first patient of the afternoon she too had a lump in one breast. There was no real doubt that this was a carcinoma, but the patient was not co-operative enough for this to be confirmed by a needle biopsy. Should a general anaesthetic be given to enable the diagnosis to be confirmed? And once confirmed would surgery or radiotherapy be justifiable? Would they prolong the patient's survival or improve her quality of life? Perhaps it would be better to do nothing, as the patient might well die of intercurrent illness without the carcinoma having caused her any trouble? In the circumstances the radio-therapist advised a simple hormonal treatment given by two tablets a day which might well cause the cancer to shrink for the remainder of the patient's life, without producing any side effects.

Clinical Judgement

In the car park the radiotherapist loaded his bag of patients' notes into his car, before the 30-mile drive back to the regional cancer centre. There was an administrative meeting that evening that he needed to attend. 'How much of what we do is really based on scientific knowledge, and how much is determined by what we believe is best, and on what is available?' he mused as he turned out of the gates of the district general hospital. 'How often do our actions mean life or death for our patients? and when is cancer treatment a matter of urgency? If we cure more "early" tumours than "advanced" ones, is that always because of prompt treatment? Perhaps the "early" cancers are those which because of their relatively non-aggressive behaviour lend themselves to long-term or permanent cure irrespective of the precise nature of the treatment or its timing? On the other hand, if I had a painful deposit of cancer in my spine, would I not expect radiotherapy immediately which would get rid of the pain, and enable me to sleep and perhaps return to work? If my wife were to develop breast cancer, would we not be distressed if treatment were delayed, even though I am doubtful whether the final outcome is affected by delay? As for clinical trials, they are fine for comparing different treatments, but they can never tell us how to treat any individual patient. That is a matter for clinical judgement.'

It was a fine clear evening and slipping a favourite tape into the cassette player of his car he swept on towards the city and his administrative meeting.

Part 5

Decision Making

Robert Lefever

The Author

Robert Lefever is a graduate of Corpus Christi College, Cambridge, and the Middlesex Hospital. He is a General Practitioner in a fully private practice in South Kensington and he is also the Director of the PROMIS Recovery Centre, a 32 bed treatment centre for all forms of addictive disease, in Nonington, Kent.

His wife Margaret works with him as physiotherapist and medical laboratory scientist in the PROMIS Unit in London, and also helps to oversee the management of the treatment centre.

They have three grown-up children, a dog and three cats. Dr and Mrs Lefever's main common interest is music.

5

Decision Making

Case 1

'Your function is to keep my husband alive until the children have finished school.' Not all patients are quite so direct in their expectations of me in my capacity as their general practitioner but this lady knew exactly what she wanted. Her husband had cancer of the intestines and it had already spread to his liver. Their youngest child was just nine years old. My chance of satisfying her demand was zero.

She came to me with absolutely clear expectations which manifestly I could not meet. My first and foremost decision was to identify her as the primary patient and fear of bereavement as the primary problem. None the less, my approach to her and her problem would only have a chance of being constructively helpful if initially I focused all my attention on her husband and his cancer. Going with the resistance, rather than fighting it, is the counselling principle involved.

Case 2

The son of an elderly woman said to me 'I expect you will tell me that my mother can be left to die in peace but that is not my view. I want to know that everything possible was done to save her, otherwise I could not live with myself.' In this case future potential guilt, rather than fear, was the motivating impulse.

Again I would need to go with the resistance, but the difficulty here is that the time scale is likely to be short and so I would have little opportunity to help the son to recognise and come to terms with his own grief reaction. The risks would come from two opposite directions: on the one hand, if I began to do the high-powered clinical investigations they could never surmount his increasing concern: on the other hand, if I went straight into talking about his own emotional involvement without first doing any clinical tests or calling in at least one specialist from the roll of the 'Great and the Good' then he would simply drop me and find specialists for himself. Furthermore, he might be in danger of finishing up with specialists who had no perception wider than physical illness. While this might be what the son purports to want, it may not be what he most needs. But the question then arises as to who has the right to decide the relative values of wants and needs, let alone the appropriate use of resources.

Case 3

'I have no doubt that I was responsible for my father's suicide when I was 15 but I have not come here to discuss that.' When I take a general medical, family and social case history from a new patient it may reveal all manner of disturbing features, but I believe that primarily, I am the patient's doctor only by invitation. Perhaps at another time the occasion for further discussion would be appropriate. Perhaps not.

Where no other patients or conflicts of issues or interests are involved, there is every reason why the patient should call the tune. I may like to believe that as a result of my professional training and experience I know best, but I am not at all convinced that this is always (or even often) the case. After all, I see only a tiny fraction of patients' lives even when they 'unburden' themselves comprehensively and especially when I may be tempted to believe that I 'know' them.

Case 4

'I need a prescription for Ritalin because I feel better when I take amphetamines and that proves that my body needs them.' The patient's doctor by invitation or otherwise, I still have the responsibility to act according to my professional understanding and beliefs ('ethics' sounds so pompous) even, and perhaps especially, when this involves directly disagreeing with a patient and refusing to take a requested action.

Case 5

The issue of who knows best for whom has many guises: 'The specialist has advised radiotherapy rather than surgery. What would you advise?' To reply that the specialist knows best — which is precisely why he or she is a specialist — misses the wider nature of the question. The patient may indeed want technical information and to a certain degree I can give it although it would be highly doubtful that any GP would have the technical understanding of the issues involved in this instance in order to be able to give a reasoned scientific response. However, behind the obvious statement of the question may be a more personal wish to share anxiety with someone whom the patient has known for a long time and who has at least some medical knowledge of the condition. Thus, in this case my function may be more interpreter, go-between and comforter than technical adviser.

Case 6

But whereas my position and that of my patients may at times be reasonably clear, there are other times when it is difficult to know where to start: 'My wife obviously needs some sort of tranquillizer or a referral to a psychiatrist' is absolutely clear and to the point but who is the patient — the wife or the husband, both or neither, and what is the problem?

Influences on Medical Decisions

The decisions I make in day-to-day general practice depend upon the patients and problems I see. The examples I have given are vignettes that every working GP will recognise in general if not in particular. But that is as far as the similarity goes. My examples were from real patients and I have a clear picture of the individuals involved: they are not identical to any other patients, nor are their situations identical to others. They are unique. Equally, I am unique. The patients and problems that I encounter are similar to those of other doctors, but my perception of any situation may be different from theirs. Each of us interprets what we see according to our own personalities as well as according to our own clinical and social perspectives. My decisions reflect me and my practice (and the geographical area in which I work) even more than they reflect any clinical medical absolutes.

The Reality of General Practice

Perhaps it is necessary to spell out the reality of general practice. The intricate decisions on precisely what diagnostic tests to do for a particular patient, or which line of treatment to follow, are relatively *infrequent* problems. The majority of my work involves common conditions and well established patterns of care. The bedrock of general practice is minor ailments: respiratory, gastrointestinal and urogenital infections, musculo-skeletal pains and trauma, skin conditions, headaches, visual problems and emotional and social mishaps and concerns of one kind or another. Every consultation has an emotional component of some form and consultations that are exclusively emotional in content may constitute up to one third of the work, or at any rate take up to one third of the total time. A further significant amount of time — perhaps a fifth of the total — is spent on general health issues: checking on raised blood pressure, diabetes and other common conditions, monitoring pregnancy and early childhood development, doing inoculations and so on. The heroics of television soap operas

certainly occur, but they are not the daily or hourly occur-
rences in real life that they need to be in order to maintain
continuing interest in fiction.

Maintaining interest in the real life situation of general
practice may become a problem for some doctors simply
because the 'sharp end' of acute medicine and surgery is so
rarely a significant part of general practice. Most commonly
when GPs see a patient in acute need we promptly refer him
or her on to hospital and often that is the end of our direct
clinical involvement, although we may be very much involved
in wider issues such as helping friends or relatives.

Those of us who maintain a love of our work do so by
becoming fascinated by what we do see rather than wistfully
recalling the days of drama and clinical rarity on the wards of
our teaching hospitals. Furthermore, as our time scales stretch
to years, we see patterns develop and families grow up and
this sharply contrasts with the focus upon minutes, days or
weeks in hospital medicine.

The Safety of Routines

Thus, the day-to-day decisions for most of my work involve
following simple, well established routines. Indeed, it is very
much in the patients' interest that I *should* follow a disciplined
routine; it is only by following my routines that I remember
what I should do, regardless of whether I am bright or tired,
happy or sad, busy or slack and so on. The safety of routines
is that they remove an important variable: me. That is not to
say that I become a robot. Far from it, it means that I am
wide awake when something does not fit the standard pattern.

At the same time, doctors will only see what they look for
and the great fascination of general practice is that no
specialist sees anything that I have not seen first. It is just
that he or she sees that particular condition more frequently
and knows more about it. But the fun of initial diagnosis or
curiosity is mine. None the less, I am happy to refer on to
specialists at a relatively early stage on the diagnostic and

therapeutic pathway simply because I believe it to be clinically responsible to do so. If a specialist does not know considerably more about a subject than I do then why is he or she a specialist?

General Practice is a Specialty

On the other hand, my belief is that general practitioners are themselves specialists. We are a very great deal more than sorting offices for hospital consultants. Only about 5 per cent of my consultations result in referral to a specialist. Most of the rest are minor ailments but, as I mentioned, at least one third of my work is the emotional work that would leave specialists — even (and perhaps particularly) psychiatrists — gasping for air. My contemporaries who have gone on to become specialists could not begin to do what I would consider to be my specialist work any more than I could do theirs.

For example, looking at the 'My body needs amphetamines' and 'My wife needs a tranquillizer or psychiatrist' cases that I gave at the start, many hospital specialists would probably be inclined simply to say 'no' to the first and 'yes' to the second and then get on with looking for what they would consider to be 'more important' or 'real medicine' work. To be simply clever and say something clinically correct, even politely and considerately rather than dismissively, to each of these patients in my examples would, in my view, be inadequate professional care in general practice. Each of these patients is a human being in just as much pain and suffering as if he or she had cancer, heart disease, or a fractured leg. Commonly when I mention to specialists in physical diseases my own interest in diseases of the human spirit they will tell me in an avuncular if not overtly patronising manner that they know *exactly* what to do for those patients — and then proceed to give me a two-sentence therapeutic remedy for an area of clinical work that has challenged me for a quarter of a century.

To refer the general population (rather than those with specific psychoses — such as those patients who believe the television watches them) to psychiatrists would change the nature of the problem: the observer alters the observed. The great advantage of seeing patients in general practice is that it *is* general: patients come with no preconceived label or sense of shame and neither do I.

Patient-centred Medicine

Thus I believe that GPs have a particular area of responsibility in managing emotional problems. This is because no one is better placed to do it or has better opportunity to develop the necessary skills, and partly because when these problems are mismanaged there may be repercussions in a whole range of medical departments for many years: appropriate management of emotional problems is preventive medicine at its most vital and, indeed, most cost-effective.

Incidentally, there are those who argue that NHS General Practitioners have neither the opportunities for training, nor the daily time, to do this form of work. This is complete rubbish. Many do it and so did I when I was in an exceptionally busy NHS practice: training and time are merely functions of organisation. Some GPs are not good at this work and may even resent it, but that says more about them than it does about general practice, the purpose and content of which should surely to some extent be defined by patients' concerns rather than exclusively by those of the medical profession.

The limit to such 'patient-centred' medicine comes when there are others better trained or placed than the GP to do particular work. In this respect I believe that a great deal of work currently done by doctors in NHS general practice could be done by trained nurse practitioners attending to minor ailments and monitoring common conditions within defined protocols. More significantly I believe that social work should be divorced from NHS general medical practice: patients' housing problems and financial problems may have great influence upon their health, but this does not mean that an expensively trained doctor is the best person, nor an expensive health centre the best place, to deal directly or indirectly with such matters.

Thus, the questions that I ask myself in any consultation are:

1. Do I know what this problem is due to, or at any rate know how to investigate it?
2. If not, who would?
3. Would the patient be better served by being referred on to someone else or by spending more time with me?

Clinical Decisions

Over the years my answers to these questions have changed. In my early years I was concerned to learn the basic clinical material of general practice and my decisions on how to spend my time and what importance to give to any particular issue tended to be slanted towards physical problems. In my middle years I became obsessed with issues of practical management: the design of health care systems and medical records, protocols for clinical management, political and social implications in the microcosm and macrocosm and so on.

Now, I suppose in my dotage having turned 50, I am content with the establishment that I run and with the clinical support of my partner and staff and with the consultant specialists to whom I refer patients. My interest focuses now on keeping my feet on the ground in basic general practice and in looking increasingly at the areas of work in which I have developed my particular skills. 'The system works: now what shall I do with it?' is the question that I find most absorbing and which I anticipate will dominate the rest of my professional life. In this respect I consider myself exceedingly privileged: I work in fully private practice and am therefore at nobody's mercy except my patients.

Thus my clinical decisions are nowadays straightforward. I have no shame whatever in admitting when I do not know what is best for a problem that I see relatively infrequently even though it may be something that is part of the basic undergraduate curriculum. For example, I have not seen an acute heart attack for several years nor delivered a baby for over 25 years. I am sure I could *somehow* manage both of these conditions but I believe that my patients deserve better than that. These clinical events simply do not occur frequently in my practice even though I do approximately 7,000 consultations each year. My decision therefore has been to let go that side of my clinical knowledge and refer on to specialist care at an earlier phase than I would have done earlier in my clinical career. Commonly in physical problems in which my knowledge is inadequate I ask my partner who, frankly, is a better doctor in this respect than I am. I do not believe that doctors can afford to be proud in pretending that we know everything: we do not.

The Value of Experience

On the other hand there are clinical as well as administrative fields in which every one of my 25 years of experience will help me. Perhaps the easiest illustration of this point would be to consider the clinical questions 'Does this issue *really* matter?' or 'Should I be *doing* something?' In my earlier years in practice everything always mattered and I was always doing something. (To his credit my partner has a much more sound judgement than I did at his stage — and even than I have now in some respects.) But now I tend to look at clinical problems with a greater awareness than previously of their wider implications: comparing my present self with my earlier self I tend now to listen more and to give advice less.

Personal Philosophical Values and Decision Making

In looking at the general issue of medical decision making, I find that it seems to me to be really a question of personal philosophical values. My days of 'how can I *fix* this patient?' are still there when clinically appropriate but they have in many ways been modified by 'how will the patient best learn to cope with this situation in future?' and 'is my personal view of any relevance?' It is not so much that I have lost confidence in myself (although I believe that is certainly appropriate in some areas of clinical management of acute physical conditions: other doctors can do that work better and I should ask them to do so). Rather, I have gained greater respect for the powers of the human body, mind and spirit to look after themselves. Perhaps people might guess from this that I believe in homeopathy, naturopathy, acupuncture and the rest of the alternative scene. In fact I do not, although I am perfectly happy for patients to believe in these things and to go to the corresponding practitioners alongside seeing me. I equate this with having different political or religious belief: it is the privilege of the patient.

My belief in the homeostatic potential of the human organism is not based upon fear of antibiotics and reverence for vitamins but rather upon scepticism for the whole charade of clinical medicine. Frankly I do not believe that patients' lives are invariably improved by medical intervention. A fair amount of what I was taught in medical school has turned out in time to be dogma or even hogwash. The management of diabetes changes with the decades and the recommendations for preventing or dealing with hyperlipidaemia (high blood fats) changes even more frequently. Psychiatry, like beauty, appears to depend upon the eye of the beholder. I do not deny that there have also been dramatic clinical advances. However, my fear is that the fact that doctors *can* do something may lead to them doing it when perhaps they *should not*.

Intervention

The obvious examples of unnecessary surgery and excessive prescription of psychotropic drugs are simply the tip of the iceberg. I am much more concerned by the general assumption that society — and the medical profession as its instrument — has the power and responsibility to intervene in all manner of areas where I believe its validity is highly suspect. The provision of state medical or social services is a specific case in point. It is *not* obvious that they are helpful: they may be harmful. They may in some instances reduce the recipients' ability and preparedness to be self-sufficient and, even more dangerous, may lead to a society that assumes that the state *is* providing when in realistic terms it is not.

The NHS is Undefined Rather Than Underfunded

The argument that the NHS would work better if it were not underfunded is also untenable; it is *undefined* rather than underfunded. It has the funds to carry out whatever specific project it wishes but it has never been specific about what is meant by 'health'. The NHS can never possibly have sufficient funds to give everything to everybody: there must inevitably - — whatever the total budget — be a definition of relative values in what is considered most important and what is not. While the NHS is undefined in its purpose it will continue to be a political football rather than specifically an instrument of health care, and those patients who need the most help (the aged, the chronically sick and disabled and the mentally sick) will continue to be those least likely to get it.

Addictive Diseases

It was largely from this awareness that I came not only to leave the NHS but also to develop my absorbing interest in addictive disease. In this particular instance what I learnt in medical school was negligible and even what I was taught was arrogant nonsense. The UK is a full 20 years behind the USA in the understanding of addiction as a disease that is not itself the fault of the sufferer but is a tendency that is probably genetically inherited through disorders of neurotransmission in the hypothalamus of the brain. While the UK continues to moralise and to ramble on about psycho-social causes and treatment, the USA has built over 3,000 treatment centres based on the principles of Alcoholics or Narcotics Anonymous. Yet still in high places in the UK the arguments are heard that the Americans are a different population from the British and that the profit motive universally dominates their health care system. Little England rules! Heaven forbid that our NHS specialists and policy makers should ever visit any of these USA treatment centres (many of which function on a non-profit basis) to find out something about treatment! Frankly, the UK provision of state services for addictive disease is rudimentary in the extreme.

From Doctor-centred to Patient-centred Medicine

Thus, my clinical career of decision making has progressed over the years from how to investigate and treat a patient's physical, emotional or social problem to how to manage a system of medical care and now to how to influence a pattern of ideas. At the same time I have progressed from initially being concerned with the medical profession, to later being concerned with my own medical practice and now to being concerned primarily with the life of the individual patient in front of me.

It might be believed that all doctors are always interested primarily in the lives of the patients in front of us. I do not believe that to be true. I believe that more commonly our interest primarily focuses on demonstrating our own professional skill. That is the way many of us were trained and it is still reflected in many aspects of professional medical culture. The gradual change from doctor-centred to patient-centred medicine has been a transition not only in my own clinical career but also more broadly within medical thinking during my professional lifetime even while technological advances multiply — and perhaps even in part as a direct result of them doing so.

So, my daily decisions have very little to do with pondering over referring patients to this or that specialist or hospital. My current range of specialists are used by me because, from trial and error, I have found that they are technically good at their job and administratively good at being readily available and at writing to me or telephoning me. Nor are my decisions laboured over precisely what diagnostic test to do or courses of treatment to recommend or prescribe: if I do not already know the answer it indicates to me that the time has come to refer the patient to someone who does.

The Reality of Decision Making: the Outcome of Cases

The reality of my clinical decision making is perhaps best illustrated by referring again to the examples with which I began:

Case 1

The lady whose husband had cancer expected something of me that I could not deliver. I told her that. I did not read up on advances in triple chemotherapy as she suggested I should. In due course her husband died and she removed her family from my care. I am of course familiar with bereavement counselling and with various helping agencies for people in her position. She was utterly determined to fight for life. I respect that. When she 'killed' the bearer of bad tidings, it hurt me but I understand that. My principal decision was to leave the specialists to their specialist field and accept that my own was not wanted.

Case 2

I put the old lady into hospital because having tried and failed to help her to live her last days peacefully at home, I felt that a battle between her son and me would be counterproductive. The private specialists totally concurred that we should do only such tests as were clinically indicated to ensure the patient's comfort. She died just the same and I suppose two somewhat cynical consequences are that I was not sued for malpractice and the son paid the hospital bills as a tribute to his own caring.

Case 3

I did not talk about the father's suicide, but my new patient has not come back to see me. My experience is that some people may want a straightforward, pill-prescribing GP rather than one who asks questions let alone one who brings tears of memory to their eyes. But however sensitive I try to be and however much I may try to respect a patient's dignity and personal wishes, I simply cannot win all of the people all of the time. For all I know there may well have been incest issues involved in this particular lady's childhood. Maybe one day she will want to talk to someone: maybe me, but I doubt it. None the less, I have not changed my standard questions.

Case 4

To the patient who requested amphetamines I explained the nature of physiological withdrawal (which is easy) and the spiritual nature of addictive disease and recovery (which is difficult) but only *after* allowing him to talk for a lot longer about his own concepts: he needed to know that he was being heard before he would listen. Even so I did not get through. This did not deter me from doing the same again next time with another patient: addiction work is certainly the most demanding work that I have ever done — but it is also the most rewarding.

Case 5

I said that I was simply the wrong person to talk to about either radiotherapy or surgery and that I had every intention of remaining the wrong person. I am not a hospital doctor, I do not have a hospital doctor's training, experience or even perspectives. Any figures that I might quote or look up would simply be from hospital doctors. What I could do was to refer the patient to another specialist to see if the second view substantially differed from the first. At the same time we talked about the bore of having the disease in the first place.

Case 6

'My wife needs a tranquillizer or a psychiatrist' has at least two obvious translations: 'I myself am having an affair' or 'She says I drink too much.' And that is where what I consider to be my specialist work begins and that is where science gives way to art.

Science Gives Way to Art

I have no idea *how* I do my counselling work. I know the standard techniques in which I have been trained (as a post graduate outside the NHS) and I know the processes that I discuss with my supervisor and with other counsellors whom I respect, but there is no exact protocol any more than there is for interpreting a piece of music. Although my approach is as disciplined as for physical conditions, I am not consciously aware of many of my counselling decisions as I make them: I simply do it my way.

Part 6

Current Practice in the Treatment of Cancer

Iain W.F. Hanham

The Author

Iain Hanham was educated at Emmanuel College, Cambridge, and completed his clinical studies at Guy's Hospital, London. He is Consultant Radiotherapist and Oncologist at Westminster Hospital which has an international reputation for pioneering the treatment of cancer.

Dr Hanham is currently involved in the restructuring of the cancer services in North West Thames and is Chairman of the Riverside Health Authority Cancer Services Committee, which is developing clinical audit. He is a member of many voluntary bodies raising funds in the independent sector for health care for the cancer disabled, particularly The Marie Curie Cancer Care Foundation.

Dr Hanham serves on The International Union Against Cancer in Geneva, and has contributed to their major publications on the treatment and long-term care of those living with cancer.

6

Current Practice in the Treatment of Cancer

Oncology is the name given to the study and treatment of cancer. The usual modalities of therapy are chemotherapy, radiation and surgery. Also involved are epidemiology, immunology and early diagnosis. A clinical oncologist is primarily concerned in the treatment of patients with cancer and may also be involved in research, if it applies to clinical problems, particularly gathering data. The speciality has gradually evolved over the last forty years with the advent of more sophisticated radiation equipment, the discovery of cytotoxic agents used in chemotherapy of cancer, and improved surgical techniques. Improved treatment has not altered the survival of many cancers over these last forty years. However, there is a clearer understanding of epidemiology, and probable causes, as a result of identification within gene structures of oncogenes, which code the neoplastic transformation in human host-cells, and are often part of the carcinogenic process.

The speciality has grown, although the number of practising oncologists remains relatively small compared to the United States. Expertise and equipment are grouped in the major centres in the United Kingdom, often meaning that patients must make long journeys for treatment, which can be particularly daunting for elderly patients. Some attempt has been made to rationalise these services, particularly in the Thames regions, using consultation and professional reviews, but many centres within the teaching districts have resisted change and amalgamation. Chemotherapy is also given on a day-care basis far from the patient's home and with unpleasant morbidity.

Trial And Error Approach

Much of oncology is palliation of symptoms, or a serious attempt to reduce the morbidity of effective but arduous treatment techniques. A recent review by the College of Radiologists (Oncology) has highlighted that many treatment regimes, particularly in radiotherapy, given for the same tumour can be very different from centre to centre. In some centres, treatment is given very quickly over several consecutive days, or only once or twice a week in much larger doses. The rationale of all this is difficult to explain scientifically to the non radiation oncologist, but reflects the somewhat trial-and-error approach to treatment that has developed over many years, many common tumours do not respond to radiotherapy but are treated in the hope they may.

Removing Restrictive Practices

As the population ages, more people will develop cancer and strain the resources of this small specialty group. Attempts are being made, however, by hospital management to unlock the restrictive manning of equipment by technicians which results, ultimately, in it being used only 8 out of 24 hours per day. These attempts include the introduction of a shift system, abolishing national pay scales, as proposed for special hospital trusts, and negotiating terms for working overtime and unsocial hours. It is hoped that more flexible working conditions will help overcome the current recruitment problem and compensate for the difficulties experienced by staff working in major cities, often in deprived areas, where many cancer centres are sited.

Labour and Revenue Intensive

Cancer treatment is labour and revenue intensive. Many procedures, such as surgical biopsy or identification of disease, may include a major operation. Histopathologists process tissue with special computer technology and radiation treatments use expensive linear accelerators which require as many as six technicians to operate effectively to treat up to sixty patients a day. Often patients have to be admitted for treatment into the acute service unit, although hostel accommodation can be used when it is available. The costs of providing counselling services for patients and relatives, and information which has to be communicated to the GP in order to deploy community care resources, must also be taken into consideration.

Furthermore, a considerable period off work for the younger age group, a period of rehabilitation, adjustments to stomas, artificial prostheses, and redefining of professional skills and working practice will all need to be considered from the point of view of economic consequences. A patient may never work again. Employers may not be too happy about some of the complications of prolonged hospital treatment and may not wish to keep the patients on their payroll. Time off work is often needed to look after a spouse and this can present further problems for the immediate family.

The American Cancer Society

There are usually many unanswered questions in the minds of cancer victims, particularly where it is difficult to be absolutely truthful about a particular diagnosis. Younger patients are denied insurance policies or mortgages and many cured patients have to adjust to disability which can affect their work. The American Cancer Society, of which there is no equivalent in the United Kingdom, is an ideal pressure group for patients and their relatives, lobbying federal government and anticipating health insurance problems including those of patients who may lose health cover if they lose their jobs because they become uninsurable due to their disease. Because the place of work and type of health care are often interlinked in America, cancer victims often become social and financial casualties, especially those who need expensive and prolonged treatment.

The British Patient

The British patient does better, except that he or she may be privately uninsured or unemployable and may need to adjust to a reduction in standard of living, unless treatment is quickly successful. The self-employed in Great Britain often have private insurance, but British medical insurance has many exclusions built into its schedules so that it may be of little use to those who are off work for a long time; if cash rebates are paid then these types of policies will *not* qualify for tax relief, in spite of recent actions by the Treasury giving private insurance tax relief to those aged over 65 years. Cancer treatment is excluded in many insurance policies because it may involve prolonged treatment and high nursing costs particularly in terminal care, which may seriously deplete family resources if the patient survives for many months. Mutual insurance is too expensive for many younger wage earners and it is often discovered at a high cost later in life that certain illnesses are excluded by the nature of the policy. Thus, doubts are created as to the private insurance sector's ability to cater for the long term sick, even though recent government legislation allows for tax relief in those carrying their policies into retirement. Unfortunately, however, these policies are often *not* designed to meet many of the problems of old age and are in effect useless for the infirm and chronically sick, who may have to rely on the voluntary charity sector for their nursing care.

Outcomes and Treatment

Many people think of cancer as an inevitably deadly condition, with mutilation, pain and unpleasant treatment. Many doctors who are not properly trained in oncology are unable to cope with patients or their relatives, but most primary care physicians (general practitioners) should be well trained to recognise symptoms of cancer even if they have little exposure to cancer therapy.

Cancer screening raises many false hopes in government that it will improve the prognosis of certain cancers. Unfortunately the facts do not support this expectation, a situation that often leads to demands for more resources.

Breast cancer can be diagnosed with mammography but in 85 per cent of cases there is a clinical mass due to invasive cancer. The other smaller groups appear as tiny areas of calcification with no breast mass, and these can be treated with simple surgical excision provided the area can be localised at the time of operation. Mammography in 50-year-olds and early 60-year-olds has been shown in one Swedish survey to increase early detection rate, and so save lives. In fact, technically, this is the easiest group to screen because the radiological images are easier to interpret; in younger women the breast has a different consistency and it is essential that any mammography is accompanied by a trained nurse or doctor's clinical assessment. Such a programme requires resources and training with a clearer public education in what can be achieved by this service, rather than allowing random and uncontrolled breast screening at any age. But the number of tumours picked up per number actually screened is very small and many have the clinical signs of breast cancer before being X-rayed.

Cervical cancer still has a high mortality but is relatively rare and may be associated with papilloma virus infection. Those identified late, as is often the case, will die early and, despite mass screening, the death rate remains unaltered.

Other Programmes

Other programmes — of safe food, giving up tobacco products, alcohol, and hazardous occupations — have been written about for many years, but without a major epidemiological shift away from preventable cancers. However, other research, such as studying the genetic sequences, may identify an important precancerous state in the patient, whose oncogene could be replaced before the disease develops; or the patient could be counselled to avoid trigger mechanisms, such as tobacco, in order to prevent its onset. This is a much more sophisticated approach than just identifying the disease in its early stages, which is the basis of most screening programmes.

The other argument is whether certain cancers are worth treating at all, even at their early presentation. Lung cancer is invariably fatal within a year, whatever modality of treatment is employed. Many clinicians electively do not treat, leaving any intervention to late symptom relief. The same applies to the commonest brain tumours, where no response is seen with complicated technological procedures.

Living with Cancer

The failure to cure cancer creates a massive social and communication problem. Hundreds of thousands of people have cancer in the United Kingdom at various stages of biological development. A few are cured, including many children and selected leukaemias and testicular tumours in adults. Patients will often be undergoing expensive surveillance while still attending school or work, with children exhibiting some retardation factors as a result of their treatment, which throws another burden on their educators.

The remainder of patients, where the disease is not yet lethal, carry on looking after families and working, but many are elderly and retired, living on their own or supporting disabled or sick spouses. Breast cancer may relapse after many years of primary treatment and will need hospitalisation for re-evaluation. At this stage of the disease the patient may need expensive chemotherapy drugs to maintain reasonable survival or to prevent pain.

Prospects

The final phases of cancer may come soon after diagnosis, as in lung cancer, and hospices and terminal care funded voluntarily have reduced the burden on local communities. There are obvious government subsidies in the form of social security payments to these institutions, yet although dedicated trained staff provide a service which is mainly nursing based, rather than acute medicine, this care is becoming more expensive owing to the rising cost of nurses' salaries and, more seriously, poor recruitment into the service.

Cancer is an expensive disease to treat. Medical audit is essential to try to correlate data on the effectiveness of treatment with the cost, because many protocols are expensive, and effective in only 20-30 per cent of patients with commoner cancers. The results of treatment are often unpredictable and need careful long-term evaluation. It is often forgotten that most treatment does not carry a cure, only a hope of living longer or more comfortably with good long-term palliative care as the clinical situation deteriorates.   T h e disease is more prevalent in the elderly so lessening its affect on gross national product in terms of work availability, but it throws considerable burdens on to the community services who have to deal with all the human suffering involved. No one has come up with a convincing argument on how to prevent the disease. Few people inherit it from their genetic make-up, some contract it from their occupations, many persist with tobacco abuse, and some may have the disease but never know because the natural history may be very slow and is often less aggressive than is often imagined.

Also Available from the IEA Health and Welfare Unit

Medicines in the Marketplace. June 1987, £5.95. ISBN 0-255 36250-1
DAVID G. GREEN, *Director, IEA Health Unit*

'If David Green's paper, the first in a series to be published by this unit, is anything to go by, a series of fascinating debates is due to follow . . . makes what could be a boring subject into a really good read.'
Nursing Standard

Efficiency and the NHS: A Case for Internal Markets?
February 1988, £4.50. ISBN 0-255 36251-X
RAY ROBINSON, *Kings Fund Institute*

'. . . the best critique so far of the internal market.'
The Independent, Guide to the NHS Debate

Acceptable Inequalities? Essays on the Pursuit of Equality in Health Care. April 1988, £8.95 (Now reduced to £4.00).
ISBN 0-255 36252-8
RUDOLF KLEIN, *Professor of Social Policy, University of Bath*
ROBERT PINKER, *Professor of Social Work Studies, London School of Economics*
PETER COLLISON, *Professor of Social Studies, University of Newcastle upon Tyne*
A. J. CULYER, *Professor of Economics, University of York*

'An interesting and provocative book . . .' *British Medical Journal*

Everyone a Private Patient. *An analysis of the Structural Flaws in the NHS and How They Could be Remedied.* June 1988, £7.50.
ISBN 0-255 36210-2
DAVID G. GREEN, *Director, IEA Health Unit*

'Everyone, rich or poor, could become a private patient', the report from the Institute of Economic Affairs says. *The Times*

Keeping the Lid on Costs? Essays on Private Health Insurance and Cost-Containment in Britain. September 1988, £5.95.
ISBN 0-255 36253-6
WILLIAM LAING, *Senior Partner, Laing and Buisson*
ROY FORMAN, *Managing Director, PPP*
NANCY SALDANA, *Head of Hospital Negotiations, PPP*
BRIAN BRICKNELL, *Personal Membership Director, BUPA*

'This short book sets a new standard of frankness about the problems of the private sector, not just in con_____ _____ of care . . . This IEA healt_ ____ _____